MENTAL HEALTH CONCEPTS IN MEDICAL-SURGICAL NURSING A WORKBOOK

MENTAL HEALTH CONCEPTS IN MEDICAL-SURGICAL NURSING A WORKBOOK

CAROL REN KNEISL, R.N., M.S.

Associate Professor, Graduate Program in Community
Psychiatric Nursing, Department of Mental Health–
Psychiatric Nursing, School of Nursing, State University
of New York at Buffalo; Ph.D. candidate in
Interpersonal Communication, State University
of New York at Buffalo, Buffalo, New York

SUE ANN AMES, R.N., M.S.

Associate Professor, Department of Adult Health Nursing,
School of Nursing, State University of New York at Buffalo,
Buffalo, New York

The C. V. Mosby Company

SAINT LOUIS 1974

TO

Kyle   *Kevi*
  Heidi   *Gregory*
    Ed   *Steve*

PREFACE

In recent years nursing educators have sought to develop integrated curricula in nursing. Although few agree on the method, most agree with the concept. We, too, found ourselves struggling with curricula that attempt to develop cultural appreciations, social awareness, and sensitivity to individual and group relationships, as well as a sound foundation for professional practice. At times the task appears too great, the faculty too divided, and resource materials too limited. We are directing our efforts toward alleviating the latter problem by writing this workbook.

Although our "integrated curriculum" calls for the placement of specialists in mental health–psychiatric nursing, in adult health, child health, maternal health, and community health settings to assist the student to utilize knowledges gained in each area in caring for patients, our experience has proved that faculty size alone makes this an unworkable—albeit theoretically sound—concept. Some have argued that any faculty member in any setting should be able to assist students to integrate concepts from all areas. Others have attempted to make a strong case for specialist versus generalist. We will not endeavor to consider the various pros and cons. What we will do is respond to a need we have identified: a practical way in which to assist students to recognize the applicability of concepts from mental health–psychiatric nursing when caring for adult patients having medical and/or surgical problems.

You will note the omission of many major health problem areas frequently included in other medical-surgical nursing workbooks. You will also note that diagnostic procedures, diet, medications, and treatments, unless very specifically related to the case in point, are absent. Religious, racial, cultural, and social aspects of patient care are limited. We trust this will not be viewed as neglectful or cursory coverage of the multitudinous influences and problems every individual may have to face in his or her daily life. We are extremely concerned about coping ability of people during periods of ill health. However, to attempt to include everything that we agree is important would make this volume unwieldy and minimize its practicality. What is important is that students become able to appropriately utilize the concepts incorporated throughout in a plan of care designed to include the whole person no matter what the religious, racial, cultural, and social aspects.

CONTENTS

PART ONE · THE PATIENT EXPERIENCING ANXIETY

1 · THREE PREOPERATIVE PATIENTS

THEORETICAL BASE

Anxiety is a general concept that explains much of human behavior. It has been described as a state of unexplained discomfort that arises from threatened loss of inner control rather than from external danger. All persons experience anxiety from time to time as an unpleasant, vague, diffuse, and frequently unexplainable feeling of apprehension, uncertainty, and helplessness that affects the ability to think, perceive, concentrate, analyze, and act appropriately.

Unfortunately, anxiety is often believed to be a specific phenomenon in individuals who are mentally ill. However, anxiety is a universal phenomenon of human existence, although persons who experience frequent and prolonged anxiety may develop complex pathological mechanisms to relieve, minimize, or hide it. It is imperative that nurses learn to recognize anxiety and fear in themselves and in their patients in order to develop effective methods for intervening into nonuseful patterns of dealing with anxiety and fear. Because all people experience anxiety, all patients, regardless of diagnosis, have the potential for being in an anxious state.

The extremely unpleasant nature of anxiety, with its resulting state of helplessness, makes anxiety difficult to tolerate. A person usually handles it by converting anxiety and the energy inherent in it into one or more patterns of relief behavior. The major patterns of relief behavior are classified as anger or aggression, withdrawal, somatization, and learning. Learning can occur only when anxiety is below the severe level. Uncomfortable and unrewarding though relief behaviors may be, they are preferable to the state of terror which is anxiety. These patterns pose problems for the person who utilizes them as well as for those with whom he comes in contact.

This case study of three preoperative patients considers the problematic nature of fear and anxiety in the face of a threatening external danger (surgery) and a threatening internal danger (isolation or loneliness, separation, or decrease in self-esteem). One way to approach the nursing care is through the framework of anticipatory fear, described by Irving L. Janis in his work with preoperative patients. Janis lays the foundation for diagnosing fear level and basing intervention on it. A condensed version, on which a number of the questions are based, follows.

3

LOW	MODERATE	HIGH
INFLUENCING FACTORS—cont'd		
Worries unproductively in a circular fashion as the result of neurotic fear.	Worries at an appropriate level markedly influenced by the information available.	Worries at the panic level when the risk of death and suffering is high and the incision is near the genital region rather than the upper abdomen or chest.
PSYCHOLOGICAL PREPARATION		
Personality tendencies that encourage evasion of "work of worrying" make the provision of information not very useful.	Stress tolerance depends in part on the external danger; therefore, it is important that control authorities make correct predictions regarding neutral or unimportant events.	Stress tolerance, mental efficiency, and ability to test reality are diminished because of hypervigilance, making it important to reduce emotional excitement to moderate level so that "work of worrying" may begin.
For those who simply need to be informed, factual statements should suffice. Combine fear-arousing statements with fear-reducing statements.	Prevent gaps in preparation through systematic efforts to give information. Give fear-arousing statements in small doses.	Give corrective information to lessen fear due to misinformation. Little benefit is expected from any program of psychological preparation if the fear reaction is a psychoneurotic one unless psychotherapy is included.

CLINICAL CASE STUDY

Bob Johannesen was somewhat relieved as he left the doctor's office. Gallstones! He could hardly believe it. Fat, fair, and forty! Well, he certainly fit those categories. He wasn't exactly looking forward to the proposed surgery—it would mean time off from work and would certainly be somewhat of a shock to his wife and children—but it was a lot better than the gnawing fear he had had for the past few weeks. Cancer—he had been sure the pain in his abdomen was cancer. He almost felt like stopping to pick up some roses for his wife—well, maybe he would do just that! Sunday would come soon enough.

Fred Schultz had repacked his suitcase for the fourth time. Being divorced had certain disadvantages, he thought—and one of them was having nobody to organize things for him. Of course, his wife probably would have forgotten something important anyway—she always did. His thin hands trembled as he refolded his pajamas. He wasn't really sure this surgery was necessary, but since he had agreed to it, he certainly wasn't going to be late. "Be at the office of admissions at 2 P.M. on Sunday," the nurse had said—and be there he would!

Kevin Kowalski was short of stature but long on enthusiasm. On this particular Sunday morning he was doing acrobatics with his 7-year-old son when he developed a sudden pain in his abdomen. Although it was sharp enough to make him catch his breath and sit down, he quickly dismissed it. His wife initially

c. high anticipatory fear—low incidence of aggressive reactions
d. moderate anticipatory fear—low incidence of aggressive reactions
e. low anticipatory fear—low incidence of aggressive reactions
1. a, b
2. a, c, d
3. a, b, d
4. b, d, e

2 Based on your observations of Fred's behavior, which of the following would you say most closely approximates what he might be experiencing?
1. low anticipatory fear
2. moderate anticipatory fear
3. high anticipatory fear
4. panic

3 Which of the following probably constituted the head nurse's rationale in recommending that the evening staff evaluate the appropriateness of individual rather than group preoperative teaching for Fred?
a. His presence in the group might inhibit both Kevin and Bob, who appeared embarrassed by his comments to them.
b. Teaching in groups may be inhibited when one participant has a significantly higher anxiety level than the others.
c. For best results, Fred should be included in a group of patients having surgery similar to his.
d. Fred may find the multiple stimuli offered in groups of people to be unsettling and contribute to an even higher degree of anxiety.
1. all except a
2. a, b, d
3. a, d
4. all of these

4 If the head nurse's suspicion that Kevin's lighthearted and seemingly unconcerned manner serves to hide his unacknowledged anxiety is correct and he is experiencing low anticipatory fear, then Kevin is likely to:
a. continue and perhaps increase his joking
b. appear unperturbed about the impending surgery
c. spend little time thinking about surgery
d. ask few questions and show little concern about preoperative preparation, the operation itself, or the postoperative experience
e. state that he does not worry about the surgery
1. all except b
2. b, d
3. a, e
4. all of these

5 Patients such as Kevin may be expected in the postoperative period to:
a. conform uncomplainingly
b. complain frequently about care

atric nurse clinician was to begin individual treatment with him that same evening.

9 It is likely that Fred's response of weeping and agitation to the surgical prep team's explanation that the skin area to be shaved included the pubis as well as the abdomen is the result of:
1. greater psychological threat when the incision is near the genital area rather than the upper abdomen or chest
2. a traumatic experience as a child involving previous genital surgery
3. lowering of reality-testing devices
4. impending psychosis

10 What are the two main purposes of the surgical skin preparation prior to surgery?

11 In the space provided, list the areas of skin and the outermost boundaries usually prepared prior to the indicated surgery. Use the figures to shade in the appropriate areas.
   a. abdominal surgery
      1. upper (e.g., cholecystectomy)   2. lower (e.g., abdominal hysterectomy)

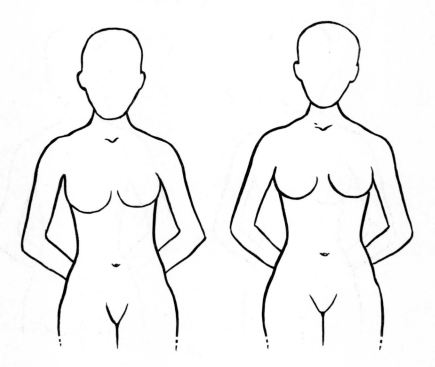

12 Why is the area to be shaved more extensive than the area actually required for the incision?

13 Fred's anxiety is indicated through both physiological and behavioral cues. List these cues as well as the others that may be indicative of anxiety.

PHYSIOLOGICAL CUES	BEHAVIORAL CUES

14 Which of the following statements about anxiety are true?
   a. Subjectively, anxiety is an unpleasant feeling.
   b. Severity of anxiety is linked with personality type.
   c. Anxiety is a state of being worried or apprehensive.
   d. Although the physical symptoms are similar, anxiety differs from fear in that there is no external threat to the person.
      1. a, c, d
      2. a, c
      3. b, d
      4. a, b, c

15 The nurse should expect that newly admitted patients such as Fred, Kevin, and Bob, whatever their diagnoses, are likely to be experiencing some degree of anxiety. Some of the factors that contribute to patient anxiety are:
   a. the hospital and its equipment
   b. fear of pain, mutilation, disability, or death
   c. fear of the unknown
   d. worries about family, job, and finances
      1. a, b, c
      2. b, d
      3. a, c, d
      4. all of these

16 In thinking of and discussing approaches in relief of anxiety, difficulties may arise because:
   1. the nursing approach has no effect on patient anxiety levels

instruction of patients scheduled for surgery began group teaching with Bob and a group of preoperative patients from other wards. Individualized instruction to be carried on later in the evening would be determined by the assessment of the specific needs of each person in the group.

20 Group instruction for preoperative patients offers which of the following advantages to the patient?
   a. He may be able to gain encouragement and support through identification with others facing a similar situation.
   b. Interaction among group members may enhance the learning experience for individual members.
   c. Active participation in the work of getting well aids the recovery process.
   d. Realistic concern in relation to impending surgery is a major goal of preoperative instruction.
      1. a, b
      2. a, c, d
      3. b, c
      4. all of these

21 Which of the following statements about planning preoperative teaching for patients who demonstrate low anticipatory fear should be taken into consideration?
   a. Evading the work of worrying through denial makes the provision of information not very useful.
   b. The nurse should give long systematic explanations.
   c. The nurse should combine fear-arousing statements with fear-reducing statements.
   d. Psychotherapy is essential during this period.
      1. a, b
      2. a, c
      3. c, d
      4. all of these

22 Using the guide below, develop a teaching program for a group of preoperative patients, including what you have learned about the physiological alterations that occur during anesthesia and surgery.

PHYSIOLOGICAL ALTERATION	RELATED INSTRUCTION
a. respiratory function	

Continued.

may be altered for better or worse, as compared with the instrumental role, which concerns itself simply with the carrying out of an assigned task. Which of the following statements in relation to expressive as well as instrumental functions are true?

    a. Performance of the expressive function decreases the likelihood of undesirable postoperative complications.

    b. In many settings a clear assignment of responsibility for attending to the patient's expressive needs is not to be found.

    c. Staff frequently tell the patient about aspects of the surgery that are important to themselves in carrying out their role but are not necessarily important to the patient.

    d. Interviews with patients postoperatively indicate that they value the nurse who performs the expressive role.

      1. a, d

      2. a, b, c

      3. b, c, d

      4. all of these

The morning after Bob had been taken to the operating suite, Fred met with one of the psychiatrists in a small conference room near the unit. After their session together ended, the psychiatrist recommended that Fred's surgery be indefinitely postponed pending outpatient psychotherapeutic treatment by the psychiatric nurse clinician and subsequent reevaluation. Fred would be readmitted for surgery when his anxiety lessened and his emotional equilibrium was in better balance. The plan for his future readmission included collaborative efforts among the surgeon, psychiatrist, psychiatric and medical-surgical nurse clinicians, and nursing team responsible for direct care.

27 The decision to postpone Fred's surgery at this time was probably based on which of the following considerations?

    a. The work of worrying is more likely to begin when emotional excitement is at a moderate rather than a high level.

    b. Fred's hypervigilant behavior is likely to further reduce his tolerance for stress.

    c. There is greater incidence of mortality in the operating room when the patient is extremely anxious.

    d. More than minimal preoperative preparation is indicated for Fred.

      1. a, d

      2. a, b, d

      3. b, c

      4. all of these

28 Fred's return home prior to reevaluation of his emotional state and readmission would certainly influence the interpersonal relationships within the family structure, which consists of Fred's aged mother and two teen-age sons. What actions would be important in assisting Fred's family with their own personal adjustment? What might be required of them in helping Fred? What are the rationales for the actions recommended?

    d. encouraging Bob to splint his incision during the deep breathing and coughing exercises
      1. a, c, d
      2. a, b
      3. b, c, d
      4. all of these

Kevin's postoperative course was not as smooth. The former happy-go-lucky ward clown began to voice angry complaints about the care he was receiving from the surgeon and the nursing team. He implied in his comments that the postoperative pain he experienced was the result of inadequate care and unfeeling attitudes on the part of the staff. The nurse responsible for preoperative instruction became upset with Kevin's response, feeling guilty despite the fact that the emergency nature of his surgery did not allow for preoperative teaching. She requested consultation with the psychiatric nurse clinician. A conference hour was set aside that afternoon for them to meet with the other nursing team members in an attempt to understand Kevin's anger and to refine the nursing care plan.

32 Hostility such as that expressed by Kevin tends to be appropriate and useful when:
    a. the energy from the emotion helps get done what needs to be done
    b. the expression of hostility lets others know and understand how their behavior affects you
    c. the degree of hostile response is appropriate to the provocation
    d. the feeling is continually repressed into the unconscious
      1. b, c, d
      2. a, b, c
      3. a, b, d
      4. all of these

33 Which of the following is the *least* important therapeutic reason for intervening into Kevin's anger?
    1. As long as anger "works," it will continue to be used and to become more automatic.
    2. Frequent expressions of anger tend to drive away the recipient of the anger.
    3. Anger often arouses insecurity and fear in personnel caring for the angry patient.
    4. There are more constructive and beneficial ways of dealing with anxiety than anger.

34 Some behavioral and physiological manifestations of anger in the adult are:
    a. harsh, loud voice
    b. increased respiratory and pulse rates
    c. glaring eyes
    d. dilated nostrils
    e. tense posture
      1. c, d, e

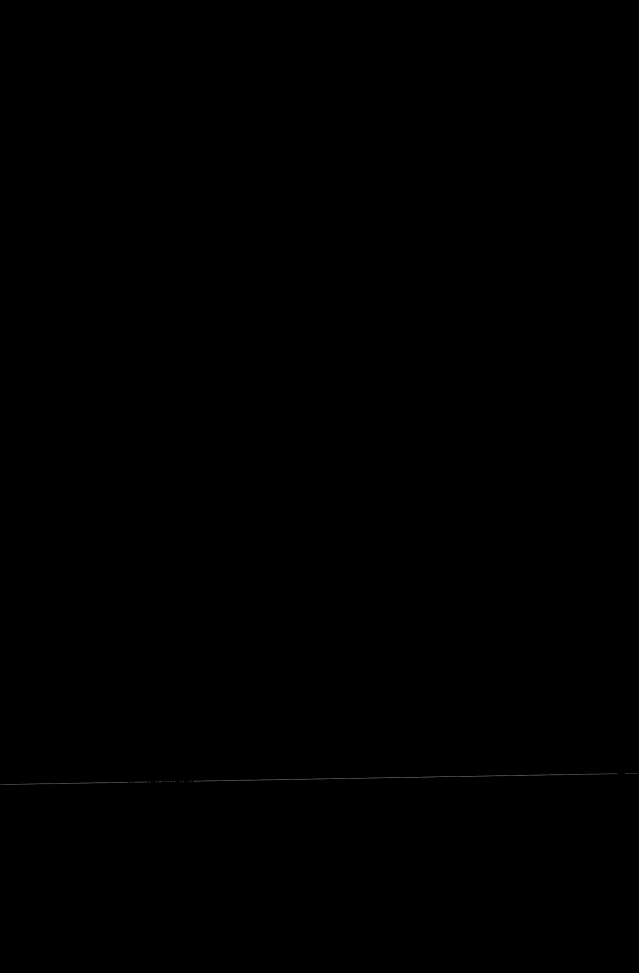

39 Guilt may be a desirable human response as long as it is appropriate to the situation. Which of the following may help in more clearly understanding such a response to Kevin's anger?

    a. Reactions to guilt may take other forms of expression, such as vague feelings of depression or feelings of inferiority.

    b. There is a universal guilt response to common experiences.

    c. Inherent in nursing are many sources for guilt feelings.

    d. Guilt is primarily an instinctive or intuitive rather than a learned behavior.

        1. a, b, d

        2. a, c

        3. b, c

        4. all of these

40 During the nursing team conference the decision was made to formulate a plan of care for Kevin through identifying the dynamics of what is happening, the rationale for intervention, the nursing intervention, and the possible outcomes of contemplated interventions. Using the guide below, formulate a plan of care for Kevin.

DYNAMICS	RATIONALE FOR INTERVENTION

NURSING INTERVENTION	POSSIBLE OUTCOMES

The consistency of the team's effective and understanding approach to Kevin resulted in a decrease of his anxiety and reduction of his anger. These measures enabled the team to redirect their focus toward Kevin's physical

2 · THE PATIENT WHO IS DEPENDENT, DEMANDING, OR DELIRIOUS

THEORETICAL BASE

Anxiety is a major influencing factor in dependent, demanding, and delirious behavior. Dependent and demanding behavior are responses to anxiety and stress, whereas delirium may be influenced by the level of anxiety.

Dependency

Dependency may be viewed as a form of regression as well as one of the first reactions to injury, sickness, or pain. People subjected to stress will tend to revert to patterns of behavior that were in some way gratifying in the past. Dependency is one of these patterns of behavior and is a fundamental human need both during the early developmental period of life and in critical and stressful periods at any time of life. Hospitalization is an example of a critical and stressful period during which physical helplessness stemming from illness is imposed. Therefore it is important to recognize the fact that sick people do become dependent and that the degree varies in relation to the physiological, intrapsychical, and interpersonal factors influencing the circumstance of the illness.

Like that of the child, the physical weakness of the adult requires the strength of others if needs are to be met. In addition, it demands that healthier persons apply their more mature and objective judgment and cognition to the events and circumstances of the dependent person's life and assume responsibility for the outcome. Paradoxically, with dependency there is ambivalence toward the benefactors, who become objects of uncritical love and admiration as well as objects of resentment because of the dependent person's weak and subordinate relation to them.

Any attempt to understand the dynamics of dependent behavior, because of the intimate relationship between the dependent person and his benefactor, must take into account the nature of the relationship between them. We know that the attitudes and behavior of nurses can limit or extend the emotional regression of the patient. For example, the nurse may encourage dependency

or to meet the demands in a way that makes her disinterest evident. In response to the unsatisfying nature of the nurse's behavior, the patient may become more demanding, thus escalating the nurse's anger and making it more difficult for her to meet the patient's demands. This may result in the nurse's further withdrawal from the patient and his greater frustration.

Another nurse may believe that the patient is manipulative and taking advantage of her and that meeting his numerous requests will be "giving in" and indulging him too much. Thus she reacts in a highly personal way, experiencing the patient's demands as a personal struggle between the two of them. Her focus then turns to what she believes the patient is attempting to "get" rather than on what his needs are or what his requests are attempting to communicate. She may believe that the patient's manner is too haughty or bossy and that he looks down on her. His manner is a threat to her self-esteem. In retaliation, the nurse may then become punishing or rejecting, thereby increasing the patient's demands.

Planning nursing intervention into demanding behavior requires that attention be paid to the following understandings. Continuing to refuse or ignore a patient's requests may make him more demanding and with some persons may contribute to withdrawal or isolation. Repeated rebuffs may force the patient to avoid relations with others. Although he may then be less demanding, his emotional distress will be perpetuated. However, interest in meeting the patient's needs tends to decrease demanding behavior. When it is not possible to meet all of the patient's demands, rational limit-setting is a useful addition to the plan of care.

Delirium

Delirium is a state of altered awareness that is frequently acute, usually reversible, and manifested by disorientation and confusion; it can be induced by a combination of physiological, psychological, and environmental factors.

The patient's degree of awareness varies considerably over short periods of time, during which he may be disoriented as to time, person, or place, as well as hyperactive, anxious, impulsive, combative, or subject to sensory misperceptions. In general, intellectual activity and reality testing are interfered with and control over inner drives is weakened. However, at other times the patient may be quite clearheaded and rational.

Delirium tends to be greater under circumstances of reduced sensory input such as that which may exist at night or in isolation units. Much of the behavior that occurs at this time is the result of the patient's attempt to make sense of his environment and the persons within it. The patient whose delirium results chiefly from an interference with the metabolic processes of the brain is more likely to experience illusions at this time—that is, he misinterprets actual external stimuli.

Much of the nursing care of the delirious patient revolves around assisting him in coping with his environment. He needs to be reoriented and helped to interpret his environment in a realistic way. The opportunities for sensory misperception should be reduced, and appropriate environmental changes should be made. Restraints are contraindicated in instances of sensory misperception

a. A decrease in the patient's anxiety will increase his dependency.
b. When immature needs are met, more mature ones will arise.
c. Unnecessary infantilizing increases dependency.
d. Attitudes and behavior of nurses can limit or extend emotional dependency.
   1. a, c
   2. b, c, d
   3. a, b, d
   4. all of these

4 In addition, a plan of care for a dependent patient should include:
a. passing through dependency to interdependency and finally to independency
b. encouraging independency by allowing the patient to do whatever he is capable of doing
c. suggesting mutual collaboration during interdependency
d. increasing the patient's individual and multiple contacts with others
   1. a, b, c
   2. b, c, d
   3. a only
   4. all of these

5 When Virgina asked one of the nurses a lengthy and complicated question about the surgical procedure, the nurse's appropriate response incorporated which of the following?
   1. a direct and factual answer
   2. the explanation that nurses are not permitted to answer questions concerning the surgical procedure itself
   3. an offer to loan her a surgical textbook that contains the answers to all her questions
   4. a brief and simple answer followed by a statement of interest in hearing more about what she's thinking and feeling

6 In subsequent conversation a period of silence ensued. The nurse made the proper decision not to interrupt the silence. This decision was based on her observation and interpretation of the silence as:
   1. stubborn
   2. rejecting
   3. thoughtful
   4. hostile

7 When the nurse entered Virginia's room during visiting hours, she found Mrs. Olmstead brushing her daughter's hair. Recognizing that such behavior might extend Virginia's dependency, how would the nurse explain the nature of dependent behavior to Mrs. Olmstead?

cerned that her demands took too much of their time, particularly since Mrs. Delacroix was allowed out of bed and was able to care for herself. Some team members verbalized anger because they viewed her behavior as rude. It became apparent that team members had begun to delay answering her call light.

10 In formulating a plan of nursing care for Mrs. Delacroix, you would recognize all of the following as true, *except:*
   1. she is manipulative, and giving in to her demands only allows her to take advantage of others
   2. refusing or ignoring her requests may make her more demanding
   3. demands may be viewed as a way of initiating and maintaining a relationship with another person
   4. demands may be related to feelings of helplessness, even though the manner may seem domineering

11 The following responses on the part of team members are likely to *decrease* Mrs. Delacroix's demands:
   a. responding to her immediately
   b. meeting the need before she must demand
   c. offering self
   d. setting limits in order to realistically meet demands
      1. a, c
      2. a, b, d
      3. b, c
      4. all of these

12 What is the rationale for each of the choices you selected in the previous question?

13 The following responses on the part of team members are likely to *increase* Mrs. Delacroix's demands:
   a. helping her to tolerate waiting by not answering her call light for increasingly longer periods of time
   b. making the observation to her that her haughty and patronizing tone of voice is inappropriate
   c. indicating sincere interest in meeting her needs
   d. being firm in the insistence that she is capable of meeting her own needs
      1. a, b, d
      2. b, c, d
      3. a, c
      4. all of these

consider staff reactions to her. Consider the reactions of team members to her when using the guide below.

DYNAMICS	RATIONALE FOR INTERVENTION

NURSING INTERVENTION	POSSIBLE OUTCOMES

The final patient presented that day was James Quinn, who was 30 years old and experiencing delirium after an appendectomy. On the evening of his second postoperative day he was dehydrated and had an elevated temperature. He addressed the nurse's aid as "barmaid" and asked to have a glass of beer. When she explained that he was in the hospital, that his appendix had been removed, and that she was the nurse's aide, he seemed to understand. However, when she returned to his room 15 minutes later to give him some fluids, Jim said: "Hi! Glad you dropped in. Let's go down to the bar in this hotel and have a drink."

20 The following statements about delirium are true.
  a. Delirium is usually reversible.
  b. Delirium is more marked at night.
  c. Delirium occurs only in persons with neurotic tendencies.
  d. Delirium impedes reality testing.
    1. a, d
    2. b, c
    3. a, b, d
    4. all of these

28 If Jim falsely believed that body organs other than his appendix were removed, and rational explanations did little to change his opinion, he would have been experiencing:
1. an illusion
2. a hallucination
3. a delusion
4. depersonalization

29 Compare and contrast the nursing interventions appropriate for patients who experience illusions, hallucinations, or delusions.

ILLUSION	HALLUCINATION	DELUSION

30 All of the following nursing measures are indicated, *except:*
1. staying with him and frequently offering water, tea, fruit juice
2. giving mouth care, sponge bath, fresh linen, cool cloth to head
3. removing or modifying such factors as poor lighting, which may stimulate faulty reality testing on his part
4. ignoring his misinterpretations of reality

31 Use the guide below to formulate a plan of care for Jim.

DYNAMICS	RATIONALE FOR INTERVENTION

Continued.

3 · THE PATIENT WHO IS DYING

THEORETICAL BASE

Increased attention is being paid within the total health care field to the processes of death and dying. The study of thanatology has become a specialty area, with journals such as *Omega* and *The Journal of Thanatology* and academic centers such as the Laboratory for the Study of Life-threatening Behavior (University of California at Los Angeles) and the Center for Thanatological Studies (University of Minnesota) devoted to it. One result of increased attention has been a significant improvement in both the quality and the quantity of care received by dying patients and their families. Another has been the recognition that those who care for the dying, nurses for example, are individuals in their own right before they become nurses. Each brings a personal and unique set of experiences to his or her professional role that influences perceptions about, and responses to, death and dying. Thus recognition has been given to the needs of nurses in their work with the dying.

Dying patients have physical and psychological needs. Physical needs are determined by the physiological state of the patient and the disease process with which he is attempting to cope. The specifics for each person need to be determined through individualized and personalized nursing care plans.

In general, dying patients may find that their senses have become less acute. When vision is less acute, dimming the lights and drawing the window shades only serve to obscure and shadow people and objects so that the dying person finds it even more difficult to order his environment. Whispered conversations to, and about, the patient are difficult for him to deal with because they withhold or reduce information and distance him from others. Hushed tones and whispering voices may be misinterpreted and become frightening. Such experiences are anxiety-provoking in nature and in a subtle way expose the patient to isolation, loneliness, and abandonment.

Exposure to isolation, loneliness, and abandonment may occur in other, less subtle and more direct ways when family, friends, and staff members limit contact or move to prevent the dying patient from preparing for and considering his impending fate despite his readiness to do so.

Figuring importantly in preparation for dying is the process of mourning—

Recently, much attention has been directed toward questions of individual right and freedom and questions of ethics and morality in relation to how one dies, as well as how one lives. Many people are coming to believe in the importance of actually having some control, when possible, over the circumstances surrounding their own death. Groups of persons have organized in an attempt to ensure the right to die with dignity when death seems imminent. Their intent is not to be self-destructive or suicidal but rather to determine to what extent artificial and/or extraordinary means will be instituted in attempts to prolong life. One example is the Euthanasia Educational Council, which has developed "A Living Will," a document through which individuals notify physicians, family members, and hospitals of their request to be allowed to die and not to be kept alive by artificial means and heroic measures.

The role of the nurse in caring for persons who are dying is extremely complex and demanding on both cognitive and affective levels, requiring the implementation of numerous skills in rendering physical and emotional care. Caring for the dying is an experience that may be emotionally exhausting for the nurse, who also must mourn the loss of a person significant in his or her professional life. The nurse is thus required to evolve a philosophy of dying, as well as a philosophy of living, to help deal with the crisis of death and the process of bereavement.

CLINICAL CASE STUDY

Ellie MacCormack spent 5 minutes giving herself a pep talk in preparation for her assignment. Mrs. Cameron, the patient for whom she'd been caring, was progressively weaker. Her condition had deteriorated steadily during the past two weeks. This was the first time that Ellie, a second-year nursing student, was caring for someone who was dying. She wondered not only whether she would be helpful to Mrs. Cameron, but also what her relationship with Mrs. Cameron's family would now be like.

During report Ellie learned that Mrs. Cameron was comatose some of the time, had an indwelling catheter and intravenous infusion, and was to have intake and output recorded. At least one member of the family had been with her constantly during these past two days. They knew there was little hope for Mrs. Cameron's recovery from a massive cerebrovascular accident and had discussed Mrs. Cameron's impending death with the physician and with other members of the staff as well.

Ellie bolstered her courage and entered the room. She spoke to Mrs. Cameron and to the two visitors, a son, Jonathan, and his wife, Linda. Jon and Linda seemed glad to see her. Although they had been able to have brief naps during the night, they looked tired. Ellie suggested that they visit the coffee shop, which had just opened for breakfast, while she bathed Mrs. Cameron. Both Jon and Linda seemed to brighten up at the thought of taking a break.

1 Ellie seemed hesitant in terms of this assignment to Mrs. Cameron. Putting yourself in Ellie's place, what might be some of her fears or concerns? What might their basis be? How might they be managed or resolved?

35

5 During the bath, Ellie put Mrs. Cameron's arms and legs through full range-of-motion exercises. What are Ellie's reasons for this activity?

6 Identify the joints and parts of the body that should be included in full range-of-motion exercises.

7 The following illustrations* portray range-of-motion exercises. In the spaces provided, identify the following:

___a. adduction   ___f. internal rotation   ___k. dorsal flexion
___b. abduction   ___g. external rotation   ___l. inversion
___c. flexion   ___h. supination   ___m. eversion
___d. extension   ___i. pronation
___e. hyperextension   ___j. plantar extension

*Modified from Terry, Florence J., Benz, Gladys S., Mereness, Dorothy, Kleffner, Frank, and Jensen, Deborah M.: Principles and technics of rehabilitation nursing, ed. 2, St. Louis, 1961, The C. V. Mosby Co.

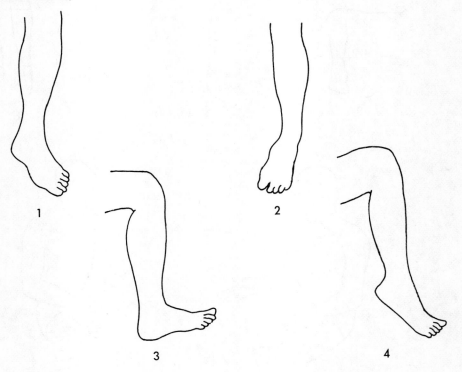

1

2

3

4

8 Since Mrs. Cameron was unable to turn herself, Ellie repositioned Mrs. Cameron on her side. The purpose of positioning a patient on her side when she cannot turn herself is to:
a. give back care
b. prevent respiratory complications
c. prevent decubiti
d. aid in circulation to skin and muscles of the back
   1. a, b, c
   2. b, c, d
   3. a, d
   4. all of these

9 Without the proper support the involved extremities of persons who have had cerebrovascular accidents tend to assume the position of:
a. adduction of the upper arm
b. forearm midway between supination and pronation
c. external rotation of the hip
d. dorsiflexion of the foot
   1. a, b
   2. c, d
   3. a, c
   4. b, d

Ellie continued to carefully observe Mrs. Cameron, who had not been conscious since that brief period when she was able to take tea and broth. Ellie noted that she felt warm and, on taking a rectal temperature, found it to be 103° F. Ellie also noted that the left side of Mrs. Cameron's face now seemed to be paralyzed, because with each respiration her left cheek was blowing in and out. Her mouth was also drawn to the left. Ellie reported her observations to Ms. Collins, the head nurse, who then accompanied her to Mrs. Cameron's room to verify the change in Mrs. Cameron's status. While Ms. Collins was examining Mrs. Cameron, she noted that her respiratory pattern was also changing and that she was now having brief periods of apnea. She immediately administered oxygen to Mrs. Cameron and sent Ellie to call the physician.

Jon and Linda were in the corridor outside Mrs. Cameron's room when Ellie returned with Dr. Franklin. Dr. Franklin asked them to wait in the conference room while he examined Mrs. Cameron. Jon and Linda had been waiting only a short time when Dr. Franklin, accompanied by Ellie and Ms. Collins, joined them. As honestly and supportively as possible, Dr. Franklin explained that the change in Mrs. Cameron's condition meant that her prognosis was grave and that extraordinary measures would be necessary to prolong her life. He suggested placing her on a hypothermia blanket to reduce her temperature, initiating feedings via nasogastric tube, oropharyngeal suctioning, and administering oxygen via nasal catheter.

Although Jon did not understand all the procedures Dr. Franklin outlined, he knew they meant additional intrusions that his mother would never want. He couldn't forget how she pulled at the catheter and the intravenous infusion,

To my family, my physician, my clergyman, my lawyer—

If the time comes when I can no longer take part in decisions for my own future, let this statement stand as the testament of my wishes:

If there is no reasonable expectation of my recovery from physical or mental disability, I, <u>MARGUERITE CAMERON</u>, request that I be allowed to die and not be kept alive by artificial means or heroic measures. Death is as much a reality as birth, growth, maturity, and old age—it is the one certainty. I do not fear death as much as I fear the indignity of deterioration, dependence, and hopeless pain. I ask that drugs be mercifully administered to me for terminal suffering even if they hasten the moment of death.

This request is made after careful consideration. Although this document is not legally binding, you who care for me will, I hope, feel morally bound to follow its mandate. I recognize that it places a heavy burden of responsibility upon you, and it is with the intention of sharing that responsibility and of mitigating any feelings of guilt that this statement is made.

Signed *Marguerite Cameron*

With permission of the Euthanasia Educational Council, 250 West 57th Street, New York, N. Y.

This document was the strongest influencing factor in Jon's decision against the use of extraordinary measures.

Mrs. Cameron died the next morning when Jon, Linda, and Ellie were in the room. Mrs. Cameron's death was not unexpected; however, it came as a shock to all of them. Although Ellie had known the Cameron family for a brief period of time, she felt emotionally close to Mrs. Cameron, and to Jon and Linda. When Linda began to cry, Ellie found herself joining in with tears of her own and grieving with them.

While Ellie cried, Tennyson's words in "The Princess" kept coming back:

> Home they brought her warrior dead;
> She nor swoon'd nor utter'd cry.
> All her maidens, watching, said,
> "She must weep or she will die."

Jon and Linda reminisced about Mrs. Cameron's kindness and gentleness while Ellie listened and occasionally added a comment of her own.

12 Ellie knew that successful grief and grieving requires crying with tears, which is typical of the phase called:
1. shock and disbelief
2. developing awareness
3. restitution
4. idealization

13 The absence of crying with tears from its appropriate phase in the mourning process may indicate:
a. excessively ambivalent feelings toward the deceased
b. the restraint of cultural patterns or expectations

Jon then began to think about Mrs. Cameron's other requests. His mother had consented to donate her eyes to an eye bank many years ago. Ellie wasn't able to answer his requests for information concerning the proper procedure to follow but stated that she could easily obtain that information for him by contacting the eye bank. However, when Ellie telephoned the eye bank she learned that Mrs. Cameron's eyes were not acceptable for donation.

Jon also asked Ellie to begin making autopsy arrangements. His mother believed that she should contribute to health research whenever possible and that autopsy was one way in which this could be done.

18 The donation of body parts and the question of autopsy are important elements in the nursing care of dying patients. Identify the factors that nurses need to understand and the actions they need to implement when attempting to be helpful to dying patients and their families.

UNDERSTANDINGS	ACTIONS
a. donation of body parts	
b. autopsy	

19 Identify the psychosocial and moral/ethical factors that would influence the attitudes of dying patients, their families, and the nurses caring for them, toward donation of body parts and autopsy.

FACTORS	LIKELY ATTITUDE
a. psychosocial	
b. moral/ethical	

PART TWO · THE PATIENT WITH ALTERATIONS IN BODY IMAGE

THEORETICAL BASE

Body image is an important determinant of human behavior because the feelings a person has toward his body are central to the beliefs he has about himself and therefore influence both his intrapsychic and his interpersonal functioning.

The body image is the concept of the shape, size, mass, structure, function, and significance of the body and its parts and allows the individual to evaluate the space occupied by the body as well as to move about freely in the environment— it is the internalized picture that a person has of the physical appearance of his body. External appearances and sensations are not the only factors that influence body image, since sensations arising inside the body, as well as the attitudes and responses of others, influence the individual's concept of his own body. In this way, body image is closely allied with self-concept, or self-image.

The body image extends beyond the physical body alone. It is known that objects of daily use such as a cane, clothes, makeup, jewelry—things that come into intimate contact with the body surface—are incorporated into the body image. The objects connected with and symbolizing professions, such as the policeman's gun or the nurse's cap, may be even more intensely incorporated into the body image, not only by the individual himself, but by the public as well. All these factors combine to form an inner mental diagram called the body image. This inner mental diagram is fluid and dynamic—it changes because of the current sensory and psychic stimuli it receives. For example, as the anatomy changes so does the body image, and as the personality changes so does the body image.

The idea of the body as "me" gradually develops during infancy. It is at this time that the child begins to conceive of himself as independent from the mother and finally independent of objects in the environment. Furthermore, he becomes able to visualize objects not only when he is with them but also when he is not, so that the word "Daddy" conjures up a mental picture quite

breast symbolizes femininity and sexual attractiveness. The mass media drive that point home in the idolization of such women as Raquel Welch, whose super-mammary endowment automatically influences the way others perceive her. In men such surgical procedures as circumcision or even inguinal hernia repair pose a threat to the body image that may be far more disturbing to the body image than such major surgery as gastrectomy or cholecystectomy. Feelings about sexuality and sexual virility are reawakened and reinforced when illness or injury threatens those parts of the body which are important to the main-tenance of the mental view we have of ourselves as men or women. One needs to be careful in recalling that the threat is great for all ages and may also be influenced by the other happenings in the individual's life space. Sometimes it is erroneously believed that surgery of the genitals or the breasts is less threaten-ing when one is "over the hill." It would be a serious error to believe that mastectomy or circumcision is less traumatic to the 49-year-old than the 29-year-old.

Another major threatening location is the face. Radical head and neck surgery or severe burns with consequent disfigurement can be devastating and require extensive alteration of body image. It is on the face that most persons with whom we interact focus their visual attention because of the importance of the face in the communication process. When the face of one person is unesthetic to another person, the reactions of both, in the immediate situation as well as in the long-term one, may pinpoint the stigmatizing nature of the body change. The interactional responses of patient, family, and friends may per-petuate a cycle of rejection and feelings of inadequacy. Consequently, most patients experience depression after facial disfigurement.

Body image misperceptions can occur after surgery. One example is the phantom experience—the sensation of feeling a part of the body that is no longer there—after surgical or traumatic removal of a body part. The phantom experience that is generally the best known is the phantom limb phenomenon, which occurs after amputation of an extremity. This experience is far more common than is generally believed. It is known that phantom limb experiences strikingly increase if amputation occurs after 4 years of age and are essentially universal after 8 years of age.

Phantom experiences occur in an attempt to redefine the lost part and to maintain the stability of the body image and its integrity. It is frightening for individuals to experience phantom sensation while intellectually recognizing the unreality of it. Other problems occur when the phantom is experienced as painful. Although phantoms are considered universal, painful phantoms are relatively rare and are considered psychopathological. Persons have described the pain by using various words such as acute, grinding, tearing, and crushing. The severity of the pain may account for the high incidence of addiction to narcotics and of suicidal tendencies among persons with painful phantom. Most forms of treatment, from cordotomy to prefrontal lobotomy, have had little effect. With increasing frequency, psychotherapy is being recommended and has been found helpful as a treatment measure. However, the time-honored tech-niques, such as encouraging the preoperative patient to talk with another person who has had an amputation, are being looked at with a jaundiced eye. Re-

47

his family, and his friends to work through their grief and thereby cope with the loss. Whether it be the loss of a loved person, a loved body part, a body function, or a loved object, successful resolution of the loss requires that grieving be completed. It may be necessary to create opportunities for some discussion of the disability, its meaning, the problem of compensating for the loss, and the possible reactions of others with whom the patient will come in contact. Attitudes of disapproval, repulsion, or rejection toward a person with a physical disfigurement or defect hinder his social adaptation. It is for this reason that nurses must recognize and then resolve their own attitudes toward, and feelings about, bodily disfigurement. To be able to assist patients and their families and friends in mutual collaboration toward a plan of care, the nurse must recognize that as a person in her or his own right, the nurse's unique beliefs or feelings can help or hinder the nursing care administered.

4 · THE AMPUTEE

CLINICAL CASE STUDY

As the evening sky flashed above him through the ambulance window, Gary Davis compared this ride with his earlier one. It left a lot to be desired, he thought, and was certainly a far cry from the freedom he felt when on his motorcycle. Although in considerable pain, Gary was aware of what was happening—and plenty worried, too! His motorcycle ride in the fresh country air had ended abruptly. The crash had totally destroyed his cycle, had damaged a tree, and worst of all had painfully and savagely torn up his right leg.

At 19 years of age, Gary was one of State College's most outstanding young athletes. His goals in life had always leaned in the direction of the health professions, but his basketball scholarship detoured those plans. Sports opened up a whole new world to him, and he reveled in the prestige and glory.

The pain in his leg refocused his attention. Gary suspected it was fractured and was afraid that he had seen protruding bone before he passed out. Had he lost as much blood as it appeared? How long would it take to heal? Would he be sidelined for the entire season? He wondered if anyone had called Janet and if she had had to call his folks. His parents could not accept his living arrangement with Janet and, in fact, had never met her, although they had been invited to come for a visit many times. He thought, what a way to bring the family together!

"Compound fracture of the right tibia with possible arterial laceration," he heard the intern say. When Gary arrived, Dr. Margaret Owens was in the emergency room and quickly assessed the situation. Gary needed to be treated for shock, and then rapid treatment for the arterial injury had to be initiated. Gary was showing signs of arterial insufficiency to the lower right leg, and Dr. Owens was concerned. She hoped manipulation of the fracture would restore the distal pulses because Intercommunity Hospital was not equipped with the kind of diagnostic services Dr. Owens believed might be necessary for Gary. Angiography would demonstrate the site and nature of the arterial obstruction, but the nearest source of such services was University Hospital, 200 miles away.

Dr. Owens saw Janet approach the nurses' station in the emergency room and heard her ask to see Gary Davis. Janet was visibly shaken. Dr. Owens immediately introduced herself and suggested they sit down to talk, explaining to Janet that Gary was responding well to treatment and was out of danger.

51

3 You are the nurse in the emergency room responsible for Gary's care. Discuss the nursing management of the patient in shock, including the rationale for your actions.

NURSING MANAGEMENT	RATIONALE

4 Which of the following are signs of arterial insufficiency in the extremities?
   a. weakened or absent peripheral pulses
   b. differences in color and temperature on comparison of extremities
   c. pallor on elevation and delayed return of normal color on lowering of the involved limb
   d. intermittent claudication
   e. tissue atrophy
   f. ulceration and/or gangrene
      1. a, b, f
      2. a, c, d, f
      3. b, c, d, e
      4. all of these

5 In observing Gary for signs of arterial insufficiency, which of the above would be relevant to his injury?

   Why?

6 Gary has been placed on antibiotic therapy for which of the following reasons?
   a. With shock there is stagnant hypoxia in peripheral tissues and wounds, which creates fertile ground for infection.
   b. Compound fractures should be treated as early as possible with antibiotics because the site is potentially infected.

53

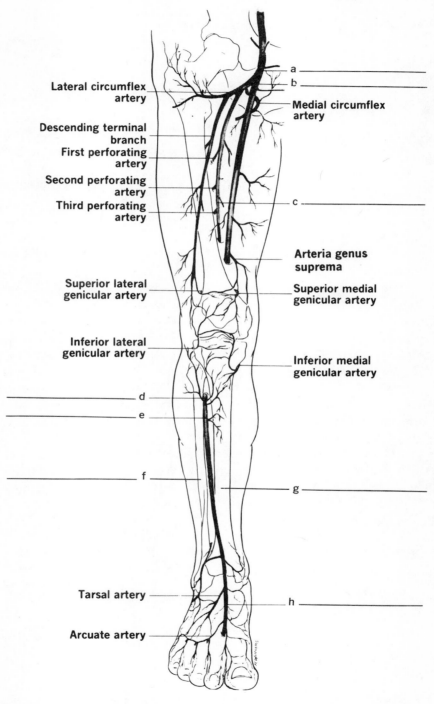

Lateral circumflex artery

Medial circumflex artery

Descending terminal branch

First perforating artery

Second perforating artery

Third perforating artery

Arteria genus suprema

Superior lateral genicular artery

Superior medial genicular artery

Inferior lateral genicular artery

Inferior medial genicular artery

Tarsal artery

Arcuate artery

a

b

c

d

e

f

g

h

Modified from Francis, C. C: Introduction to human anatomy, ed. 6, St. Louis, 1973, The C. V. Mosby Co.

b. transection

Janet spent 3 anxious hours waiting in the room on the surgical service
to which Gary had been assigned. The evening nurse was very supportive and
called the recovery room to inquire whether Gary had been admitted. "Still in
surgery," was the response. After giving her report to the night shift, the evening
nurse invited Janet to accompany her to the employees' cafeteria for a snack.
Janet was grateful for the break and, feeling very hungry, ate a substantial
meal. An operating room nurse going off duty joined them and, learning of
Janet's concern over Gary, explained that there had been some complications
but all was going well and Gary would be in the recovery room shortly. According to hospital policy, she explained, he may have to be there all night and
suggested that Janet go home and rest. Janet returned to the unit, told the night
nurse where she could be reached, explained that Gary's parents were on their
way, and went home.

Early the following morning Janet arrived at the hospital, followed shortly
by Gary's parents. Janet's meeting with Mr. and Mrs. Davis was not at all as
traumatic as she feared it would be. The three of them were caught up in their
concern for Gary, which overshadowed any interpersonal problems that might
have existed. Dr. Blake asked to be notified as soon as the Davises arrived and
requested a meeting with them in the conference room. Janet remained with
Gary while Dr. Blake explained the situation to the Davises. After discussing
the nature of Gary's injury and the surgical intervention, Dr. Blake stated:
"We have taken care of the fracture but are still concerned about the circulation
to Gary's lower leg and foot. The nursing staff is checking the circulation in
Gary's right foot every half hour and will alert me to all changes. He's doing
well otherwise. However, this is a small hospital and we're not equipped for the
sophisticated diagnostic and surgical procedures that might be necessary should
Gary's circulatory problems worsen. Dr. Owens, the intern who assisted me
with Gary's surgery, suggested transferring Gary to University Hospital. I
consulted with Dr. Sarah Kahn, a vascular surgeon there, at the time I operated
on Gary. She was very helpful and has an excellent reputation. How do you
feel about the possibility of transferring Gary to University Hospital?"

After further discussion with Dr. Blake and consideration of the pros and
cons, the Davises concurred and plans were made for Gary's transfer to University Hospital by ambulance.

10 You are the nurse responsible for monitoring the circulatory changes in
Gary's lower leg and foot. What are the nursing actions involved in this
responsibility?

somehow reduce the level of feeling experienced by the patient. The nurse has, in some way, implied that the patient need not feel the way he does.

___d. A response indicating that the nurse's intent is to teach the patient about his problem, its meaning, and his feelings. The nurse verbalizes in an obvious or subtle way what the patient with the problem thinks, feels, or experiences.

___e. A response indicating that the nurse's intent is to seek further information to promote further discussion along a certain line. The nurse has, in some way, implied that the patient would profit from developing a point, discussing it further, or going on to another, more profitable topic.

15 The nurse's statements from question 11 are repeated below. Match each statement with the appropriate type of response.

Type of response
1. evaluating
2. interpreting
3. probing
4. reassuring
5. understanding

Nurse's statement
___a. "Worrying so much only upsets you more. Let's wait to see what happens."
___b. "I don't notice any changes. It seems the same to me now as it did before."
___c. "You're really worried about the circulation in your leg. To you it seems to be getting worse."
___d. "When people seem as concerned as you are, it is evidence of anxiety. What about the condition of your leg makes you so anxious?

16 When Gary and Janet learned that Gary was to be transferred to University Hospital, Gary appeared startled but silent while Janet burst into tears and sobbed, "He's going to lose his leg, isn't he?" Write down what you would have said, assuming you wanted to respond with each of the five types of intentions.

a. evaluating _____

_____

_____

_____

b. interpreting _____

_____

_____

and could not accept Dr. Kahn's statement that everything possible had already been done to save Gary's leg. Dr. Kahn asked Charles Lambert, the head nurse on the orthopedic unit, to join them. Both Dr. Kahn and Mr. Lambert listened patiently while the Davises verbalized their feelings and frustrations. Finally Mrs. Davis began to ask some questions: "Who will tell Gary?" "When does it have to be done?" "What will it mean?" Mr. Davis interrupted, saying: "Gary will need help with this. Sports are so important to him; he'll be totally demoralized. How can we help him to adjust to an amputation?"

Dr. Kahn and Mr. Lambert remained with the Davises for nearly an hour. It was decided that Dr. Kahn and Dr. Nathan Cole, the orthopedist who would perform the surgery, should talk with Gary immediately. "Janet should be with Gary when he is told," Mrs. Davis said. "They are very close, and he would want it that way."

19 Consider both the advantages and disadvantages of Janet's presence when Gary is told of the necessity for an amputation.

ADVANTAGES	DISADVANTAGES

20 It seems as though Gary's parents and the staff are collaborating in making a decision regarding Gary. What other recommendations do you have concerning who should participate in the decision-making process and why?

21 Who else might be helpful in assisting Gary to prepare for surgery involving extensive body alteration?

22 Gary's immediate response to the news of his impending surgery was one of anger. However, when Mr. Lambert, the head nurse, reentered Gary's room, he found Gary alone and crying. What factors might influence Mr. Lambert's response to Gary?

to be able to close the wound with a flap-type procedure. However, because of the trauma and the uncertainty of the internal condition of Gary's leg, he left the option open for a guillotine procedure.

25 The decision regarding the level at which a leg is amputated depends on which of the following factors:
   a. complete removal of the diseased tissue
   b. sufficient circulation to the remaining limb
   c. a stump that allows for satisfactory fitting and functional movement of the prosthesis
      1. a, b
      2. a, c
      3. b only
      4. all of these

26 Define the two types of operative closures for amputation and the rationale for each.

DEFINITION	RATIONALE
a. closed or flap type	
b. open or guillotine type	

27 In addition to the expected preoperative teaching for any surgical patient, Gary should be taught which of the following?
   a. flexion and extension of arms while holding weights
   b. repositioning with the aid of an overhead trapeze
   c. seated arm-pushing body raises
   d. active exercise of the unaffected leg
      1. a, c
      2. b, c, d
      3. b, d
      4. all of these

28 Give the rationale for each of the options you selected.

29 A pint of blood was administered to Gary in the preoperative period, and several pints were ordered to be available during surgery. The nurse must be alert for certain adverse reactions to the transfusion of whole blood. The fol-

Which of the following are nursing responsibilities?
a. requesting side rails, trapeze, and footboard for the patient's bed
b. assisting the patient to the prone position frequently for 15-minute intervals (usually after 24 hours postoperatively)
c. encouraging frequent change of position
d. reemphasizing the importance of the exercises taught preoperatively
   1. a, b
   2. b, c, d
   3. a, c, d
   4. all of these

34 Give the rationale for each of the options you selected.

35 After the initial dressing change, the nurse may be changing the stump dressing p.r.n. Discuss the nursing responsibilities involved in this activity.

36 Later in the postoperative period a compression bandage is applied to the stump. Explain the nursing responsibilities involved in applying the compression bandage and the rationale for each nursing action.

NURSING RESPONSIBILITIES	RATIONALE
a. mid-thigh	
b. mid-calf	

Gary's progress was satisfactory during the postoperative period. His incision healed well, and he was soon able to transfer into and out of a wheelchair with minimal assistance. The physical therapist who initiated crutch walking

40 Patients such as Gary who have had time in the preoperative period to prepare themselves for amputation usually respond well psychologically in the postoperative period. What postoperative problems can you foresee in patients who have not had this time to prepare prior to the surgery?

41 Health teaching in preparation for discharge is a responsibility of the nurse. What health teaching would you undertake to assist Gary in optimal adjustment physically and emotionally to home and community? Include rationale.

HEALTH TEACHING	RATIONALE

REFERENCES

Blake, Florence G.: Immobilized youth: a rationale for supportive nursing intervention, American Journal of Nursing **69:**2364-2369, Nov., 1969.

Bosonko, Lydia A.: Immediate postoperative prosthesis, American Journal of Nursing **71:**280-283, Feb., 1971.

Brown, Florence: Knowledge of body image and nursing care of the patient with limb amputation, Journal of Psychiatric Nursing **2:**397-409, 1964.

Child, Judy, Collins, Douglass, and Collins, Janis: Blood transfusions, American Journal of Nursing **72:**1602-1605, Sept., 1972.

Corbeil, Madeline: Nursing process for a patient with a body image disturbance, Nursing Clinics of North America **6:**155-163, March, 1971.

Griffin, Winnie, Anderson, Sara J., and Passos, Joyce Y.: Group exercise for patients with limited motion, Amerian Journal of Nursing **71:**1742-1743, Sept., 1971.

Jordan, Helen S., and Cypres, Robert M.: All-around care for the leg amputee, Nursing '74 **4:**51-55, April, 1974.

Kolb, Lawrence C., Frank, Ludwig M., and Watson, E. Jane: Treatment of the acute painful phantom limb, Proceedings of the Staff Meetings of the Mayo Clinic **27:**110-118, March 12, 1962.

Leonard, Beverly J.: Body image changes in chronic illness, Nursing Clinics of North America **7:**687-695, Dec., 1972.

Roach, Lora B.: Assessment: color changes in dark skins, Nursing '72 **2:**19-22, Nov., 1972.

Thorman, George: Cohabitation: a report on couples living together, Futurist **7:**250-253, Dec., 1973.

Ujhely, Gertrud B.: When adult patients cry, Nursing Clinics of North America **2:**725-735, 1967.

2. "It seems as though you are concerned about your health and the outcome of your surgery."
3. "Oh, no, there are quite a few vacant hospital beds."
4. "I'm sure everything will be all right. Try to get some rest and don't worry about it."

3 What was your rationale for selecting the appropriate response?

4 What was your rationale for not selecting each of the remaining responses?

5 Beth later stated that she had not let her children know of her hospitalization and the proposed treatment, saying: "I haven't told them the bad news. They're both studying so hard for final exams." One appropriate response at this time might be to say:
1. "This sounds like a difficult situation for you. Let's explore it together and see what might be said or done."
2. "I think you should break the news to them now. Your immediate problem is the important one. They can always ask to take exams at another time."
3. "It isn't fair to exclude part of your family from a vital or critical incident in your life."
4. "That's good. It's wise to protect them from worry since nothing's definite anyway."

6 What was your rationale for selecting the appropriate response?

7 What was your rationale for *not* selecting each of the remaining responses?

Dr. Hansen visited Beth in her room shortly after her admission to the hospital. He explained to her the various kinds of surgical procedures currently

DEFINITION	ULTIMATE APPEARANCE	PROGNOSIS
c. subcutaneous mastectomy		
d. simple mastectomy		
e. radical mastectomy		

9 Recognizing that surgical alteration of body appearance may have profound psychological significance for the individual, what factors might influence Beth's decision concerning the extent of the surgery she will allow to her breast?

10 Since Beth has already discovered the lump in her breast, why was a mammogram ordered?
   a. It is an adjunct in diagnosing carcinoma of the breast.
   b. It can be a substitute for breast biopsy.
   c. It may serve as a comparative tool after surgery.
   d. It is the only positive diagnostic test for breast cancer.
      1. a, c
      2. b, c
      3. a, d
      4. all of these

11 In considering the location of surgery and the type of dressing Beth may

talked a while longer about the meaning the surgery might have to Beth and Jim and the children, as well as its influence on their interpersonal relationships.

15 Consider the impact of Beth's radical mastectomy on Beth, Jim, Debbie, and Carl from two frames of reference:
  a. the possible meanings of the surgical alteration of body image to each member of this family
  b. the possible influence of the surgery on the interpersonal relationships of individual family members as well as on the family unit itself

POSSIBLE MEANINGS OF BODY IMAGE ALTERATION	POSSIBLE INFLUENCE ON INTERPERSONAL RELATIONSHIPS

16 What are the factors that might be included in a consideration of the possible meanings and influences that body-altering breast surgery might have on Beth's interpersonal relationships with friends and relatives other than the immediate family?

17 When Beth entered the recovery room, the paramount concern of recovery room personnel was:
  1. keeping Beth free of pain
  2. maintaining a patent airway
  3. checking Beth's dressing for drainage
  4. maintaining fluid and electrolyte balance

18 Why did recovery room personnel keep a close watch on Beth's vital signs?
  a. Pulse and blood pressure are the best indicators of circulatory changes that could result from anesthesia and blood loss during surgery.
  b. Respirations tend to be more shallow because of the pressure dressing.
  c. An increase in pulse rate and a drop in blood pressure could indicate hemorrhage.
  d. Elevated temperature could indicate wound infection.

73

23 Ensuring proper wound healing is an important aspect of nursing care. What will you want to consider in caring for Beth's wound drainage system to provide the optimum environment for wound healing?

a. avoiding kinks in the tubing that will cut off suction
b. after emptying the drainage, reestablishing the negative pressure by compressing the unit
c. maintaining proper asepsis when emptying the drainage
d. clamping the tubing prior to emptying and compressing the Hemovac unit
e. instructing Beth to avoid lying on or putting tension on the tubing

    1. a, b, c
    2. b, c, d
    3. a, d, e
    4. all of these

24 Beth was "dangled" at the bedside and then assisted to a standing position that same evening. The nurses and Jim encouraged Beth to take a few steps and then assisted her back to bed. As a nurse in this situation, how would you carry out this activity in the safest and most comfortable manner for Beth and yourself?

25 What is the rationale for ambulating Beth at this time and in this manner?

26 Within 24 hours after surgery, Dr. Hansen instructed Beth to begin exercising her right hand and arm. Initial exercises the nurse can encourage Beth to perform are:

a. flexing and extending the fingers
b. flexing and extending the wrist
c. flexing and extending the elbow
d. gradual abduction of the arm
e. grasping the right wrist with the left hand and slowly raising the arm upward

    1. a, b, c
    2. b, d
    3. a, c, d
    4. all of these

27 Exercise of the affected arm is important soon after surgery in order to:

a. prevent limited range of motion and contracture formation

ing the incision for the first time. How would you support Beth during this experience?

One evening, just before visiting hours, Beth asked the nurse what kinds of material she could put into her bra to make her look more "normal" in the very feminine robe Jim had given her. The nurse explained that Beth should not wear a bra until the incision was completely healed. They then discussed the prosthetic devices that were available for women after mastectomy. Beth was very much interested in what the nurse had to say and immediately began to take greater interest in her personal appearance by fussing more with her hair and applying makeup before Jim arrived.

32 What information would be important for Beth to have about wearing a brassiere and breast prosthesis?

33 Beth stated that she sometimes felt "off balance" when she walked. How would you explain this phenomenon to Beth?

34 Identify the physical and psychological elements that would encourage Beth's social reintegration and increase her coping abilities in the postoperative period.

PHYSICAL	PSYCHOLOGICAL

35 Many people who, like Beth, have had surgery for cancer have concerns about its recurrence. What are the possible ways in which these concerns could affect her social reintegration and coping abilities in the future?

EXPLANATION*	ILLUSTRATION*	RATIONALE

1. Lie down. Put one hand behind your head. With the other hand, fingers flattened, gently feel your breast. Press ever so lightly. *Now examine the other breast.*

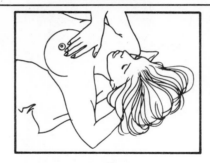

2. This illustration shows you how to check each breast. Begin where you see the *A* and follow the arrows, feeling gently for a lump or thickening. *Remember to feel all parts of each breast.*

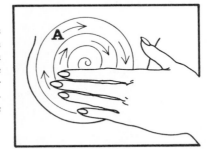

3. Now repeat the same procedure sitting up, with the hand still behind your head.

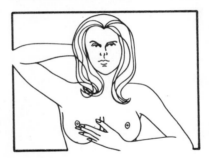

*From A breast check, New York, 1971, American Cancer Society, Inc.

41 The nurse took advantage of Beth's interest in breast self-examination to offer information concerning thermography.

a. Define thermography.

b. What is the relevance of this information for Beth and Debbie?

42 During Beth's postoperative visit to Dr. Hansen's office, Mrs. Cummings will be alert to determine whether Beth has unresolved feelings or concerns relating to the body image alteration. Which of the following would indicate problematic adjustment?

a. frequent joking about her physical appearance and the prosthesis

6 · THE PATIENT WHO IS BURNED

CLINICAL CASE STUDY

Rita Wilson, a senior nursing student, was about to spend several weeks at the burn treatment center in an independent study project. Her father, a fireman, was instrumental in stimulating her interest toward nursing as a career, and now, when she had a choice to further explore a specialty area, she selected the care of patients with burns. It was on that first day that Sally Carson was admitted.

Sally had been barbecuing spareribs on her outdoor grill when the explosion occurred. The gas company was still investigating the cause of the explosion while Sally fought for her life in the burn treatment center. She sustained second- and third-degree burns over the entire upper portion of her body, including both arms. As Rita was undergoing her orientation to the burn unit, she found it hard to ignore the activity surrounding Sally Carson. She heard that Sally was in shock, that a tracheotomy and venous cutdown had been performed, and that an indwelling catheter had been inserted. She wondered about this girl, not much older than herself, whose face had been so damaged. "How will she cope?" thought Rita. "I'm not sure I'd be able to."

After several days of orientation to the care of the burn patient, Rita asked to be assigned to the care of Sally Carson. By this time Sally's condition was somewhat stabilized, she was in a CircOlectric bed, and active management of her burns was taking place.

1 Discuss the immediate emergency care of a burn patient, using the guide below.

ASSESSMENT OF PROBLEMS	NURSING ACTION

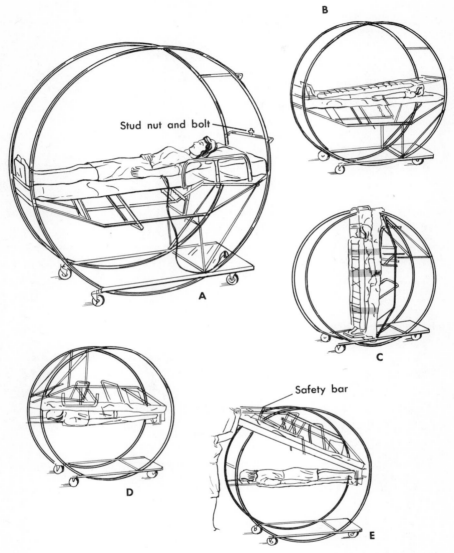

CircOlectric bed. **A,** The patient is in back-lying position, with her hips centered at the gatch. The footboard is adjusted to prevent her from sliding downward during transfer. The pillow from her head is used to pad her legs and knees. A sponge rubber face mask is applied to protect the face. **B,** The anterior frame is installed and locked in place with a stud nut and bolt. **C,** After telling the patient which way she will turn, the nurse rotates the bed electrically. Safety straps are necessary if the patient is unable to control her arms. **D,** The posterior stud nut is removed from the head of the frame, and the safety bar is pulled forward to disengage the posterior section. **E,** The posterior section is raised high overhead and locked into the circle frame with the safety bar. (Courtesy Stryker Corporation, Kalamazoo, Mich.; from Dison, N. G.: An atlas of nursing techniques, ed. 2, St. Louis, 1971, The C. V. Mosby Co.)

1. a, b, c
2. b, c, d
3. a, d
4. all of these

9 Approximately three to five days post-burn, fluids return from the tissues of the burn area to the vascular compartment. Which of the following nursing observations will give evidence of this phenomenon?
a. increased urinary output
b. profuse diaphoresis
c. reduced local edema
d. cessation of nausea and vomiting
   1. a, b, d
   2. a, c
   3. b, c, d
   4. all of these

10 Sally was weighed each morning so that estimates of fluid loss and accurate replacement therapy could be continued. Weighing a patient such as Sally may be problematic. Discuss the problems you can foresee and identify the resultant nursing actions.

PROBLEM	NURSING ACTION

11 The nurse has many responsibilities in maintaining the intravenous route of infusion. What should nurses know to give the best care to a patient receiving intravenous fluids?

12 In caring for burn patients, the urinary output is an important index of the patient's response to fluid replacement therapy. An indwelling catheter is inserted into the bladder for accurate hourly monitoring of urinary output. What are the nursing responsibilities involved in the care of this catheterized patient?

d. Systemic antimicrobial medications are prevented from reaching the wound by damage to local blood vessels and stasis of circulation.
   1. a, b, c
   2. b, c, d
   3. a, d
   4. all of these

16 There is considerable difference of opinion concerning the proper treatment of second- and third-degree burns. However, there is no disagreement about the importance of strict aseptic technique when wound care is provided and dressings are changed. What are the important nursing considerations in maintaining proper aseptic technique in the care of burns?

17 The dressing change may be very painful and anxiety producing for the patient. What nursing measures can be employed to reduce this pain and anxiety?

Rita's first few days of caring for Sally were completely frustrating, and she found herself totally immersed in the physical aspects of care. The dressings, the tracheotomy, the catheter, the repositioning, the intravenous infusion, and the institution of oral fluids required more time than the 8-hour shift allowed. Rita left the unit each day feeling like a robot instead of a human being. She recognized the importance of good physical care but felt that although Sally was progressing physically, her many psychological needs were not being considered.

Rita had been trying to piece together a portrait of Sally to help her understand the fears and problems she might have both now and later. Rita learned that Sally had a 5-year-old daughter who was being cared for by a neighbor since the accident. Mrs. Carson, Sally's mother, had been called and asked to come in to give some statistical information about Sally. Mrs. Carson, however, would only consent to giving the data by telephone. Only the neighbor evidenced concern for this young woman since her hospitalization. "Thank goodness, Sally has been reassured about the care of her little girl," Rita thought. "Parenthood must be an overwhelming responsibility, especially when you are a single parent, as Sally seems to be."

Rita had seen Sally's face without her dressings on two occasions. The experience was a shock to her, and she knew it would be more of a shock to Sally. "She must be wondering what she looks like," Rita thought. "How can we help her cope? What can we do to help her little girl adjust?"

munication? If not, why not? If so, give your rationale and suggestions for how this might be accomplished.

24 Small amounts of oral fluids were offered to Sally as soon as active bowel sounds were heard. Nutritional management of a burn patient depends on:
   a. an understanding of the protein losses in the early post-burn period
   b. an understanding of the caloric expenditures of the body in the early post-burn period
   c. early treatment of gastrointestinal disturbances such as paralytic ileus or stress ulcers
   d. continuing efforts to stimulate appetite and meet individual patient food preferences
      1. a, b, c
      2. b, c, d
      3. a, d
      4. all of these

25 Sally found eating to be an unpleasant chore. She had great difficulty feeding herself because of the arm and hand dressings. One day when Rita was attempting to assist Sally with her lunch, Sally stated: "What's the use? I'm wasting away to nothing anyway. Just leave me alone." Using the guide below, assess this situation and formulate an initial verbal response based on your assessment.

DYNAMICS	RATIONALE FOR INTERVENTION

INITIAL VERBAL RESPONSE	POSSIBLE OUTCOMES

BODY PART	PROPER POSITION	COMMON CONTRACTURE COMPLICATION	NURSING INTERVENTION TO PREVENT CONTRACTURES
b. shoulder			
c. elbow			
d. wrist			
e. fingers and thumb			

32 Define the following terms:

a. eschar

b. escharotomy

c. granulation tissue

some hesitancy about a visit from her mother and daughter, she agreed that it was important for a staff member to visit them and assess the situation.

The psychiatric and pediatric nursing clinical specialists met with Rita and the staff of the rehabilitation unit to assist in formulating a plan of care based on additional information gathered during the home visits.

33 Identify the physical and psychological elements that would encourage Sally's social reintegration and increase her coping abilities during the rehabilitative period.

PHYSICAL	PSYCHOLOGICAL

34 What actions would be important in assisting Sally's daughter and mother with their own personal adjustment? What might be required of them in helping Sally? What are the rationales for the actions recommended?

NURSING ACTION	RATIONALE

35 During their conference together, Rita, the clinical specialists, and the rehabilitation unit staff formulated their plan of care for Sally. On the following guide, identify the short-term and long-term goals, the rationale for these goals, and appropriate nursing actions.

7 · THE PATIENT UNDERGOING PROSTATECTOMY

CLINICAL CASE STUDY

E. Jarrett Haynes, executive vice-president of a large eastern bank, sat quietly in his office awaiting a telephone call. Dr. Edward Morgan, his friend and urologist, had told him that the test results would be back today, and he found it difficult to concentrate on anything else. The phone buzzed, interrupting his musings, and Dr. Morgan came on the line. "Don't worry about a thing, Jerry," he said after some initial pleasantries. "You have an enlarged prostate gland, which is fairly common in your age group. I'll schedule you for surgery next week, and you'll be as good as new." Dr. Morgan added a few instructions about reporting to the hospital and signed off, saying, "We'll have you back to your tennis game in no time."

His tennis game was not of major concern to Jarrett Haynes, but his masculinity was. Sixty-two didn't seem old to him, and since his marriage to Karen three years ago, he felt and looked younger than ever. Could he discuss with Ed Morgan, a good friend for some years, his concerns about his ability to perform sexually after surgery? He thought it doubtful, since he hadn't even been able to ask about the possibility of malignancy. He didn't understand how Ed could pass off this surgery so blithely.

Mr. Haynes had been a widower for twelve years. He and Lucille, his first wife, had four children, all of whom were grown now and married, with children of their own. His years alone were difficult ones in which he missed the loving companionship he had known with Lucille.

When Karen came into his life he felt like a young man again. She was a vice-president in his bank, 35 years old, single, intelligent, outgoing, and respected by all who knew her. They both anticipated that their age difference might be problematic, particularly in a few more years when he would be in his seventies and she in her forties. Although this subject was the focus of many conversations between Karen and Jerry, they finally decided to marry. Mr. Haynes had not anticipated succumbing to age so soon and was particularly concerned that the nature of his problem could curtail his sex life, which had given him so much pleasure in the past three years.

That evening before dinner Jerry told Karen of his conversation with Dr.

OPERATIVE APPROACH	ADVANTAGES	DISADVANTAGES
b. suprapubic prostatectomy		
c. perineal prostatectomy		
d. retropubic prostatectomy		

4 The selection of the surgical approach for prostatectomy is made on consideration of which of the following factors?
   a. age of the patient
   b. size of the prostate gland
   c. location of the prostate gland
   d. overall condition of the patient
   e. presence of associated diseases
      1. a, b, c, d
      2. a, d, e
      3. b, c, e
      4. all of these

5 In diagnosis of prostatic problems, of what value is the rectal examination?

6 Prostatic massage is often done by the urologist to obtain prostatic secretions. Of what value is laboratory analysis of prostatic fluids?

7 In assessing the overall health of the genitourinary tract, various diagnostic

9 For proper asepsis in catheterization of a male patient, which of the following are important?

   a. retraction of the prepuce and cleansing of the glans with a mild antiseptic

   b. use of sterile containers in collecting and transporting the specimen

   c. sufficient amounts of sterile lubricating jelly to lessen trauma to the urethra

   d. use of sterile gloves or sterile forceps to insert the catheter

      1. a, b, c   3. a, d

      2. b, c, d   4. all of these

10 To prevent infection of the urinary tract preoperatively, what measure can you think of that should be suggested to Mr. Haynes?

   1. decreasing sexual activity

   2. increasing oral fluid intake

   3. checking urine q.i.d. for sugar and acetone

   4. measuring urinary output

In the meantime, Mr. Haynes's symptoms became increasingly annoying. He was experiencing urgency and frequency both day and night and noticed hesitancy in initiating his urinary flow along with a decrease in the force and size of the urinary stream. He greatly feared that he would be incontinent at some inopportune moment. As his symptoms increased, his reluctance about surgery decreased.

The conference with Ed Morgan and Dr. S. R. Raman was reassuring to both Karen and Jerry Haynes. They both accepted the necessity of surgery and were pleased to learn that Dr. Raman was to perform the surgery with Dr. Morgan's assistance. The four of them discussed the variety of surgical procedures available and decided that suprapubic prostatectomy offered the best urinary results as well as maintenance of sexual potency. The fear that a malignancy might be present was reduced when Ed Morgan discussed the findings of the rectal examination with Jerry Haynes. "I was not able to palpate a nodule when I did the rectal examination and thus feel quite certain that you do not have cancer of the prostate," Ed Morgan stated. "The cystoscopic examination and intravenous pyelogram demonstrated no damage to the kidney, ureters, or bladder from retention of urine. However, the fact that residual urine was present is of concern because cystitis and ascending infections of the urinary tract can lead to severe chronic problems. And, of course, your discomfort will increase as the prostatic enlargement results in greater obstruction of the bladder neck." As Dr. Morgan explained, he pointed to the anatomical chart of the male genitourinary tract.

Before Mr. and Mrs. Haynes left the doctor's office, Ms. Yates, the office nurse, discussed with them the admission procedure to the hospital and the preoperative preparation Mr. Haynes would undergo. She explained exercises for prevention of postoperative respiratory and circulatory complications and gave them an instruction sheet for practicing the exercises at home. She shared with them what might be expected after surgery and stated that she would visit Mr. Haynes the day before his surgery to answer any questions he or Mrs.

15 Mr. Haynes experienced considerable discomfort in his first 48 postoperative hours because of bladder spasm. What nursing measures can be utilized to decrease this discomfort?

16 Early ambulation is important for prevention of many possible postoperative complications. What urinary tract complication is common after periods of immobility?

What problems could occur as a result of this complication?

Mr. Haynes progressed rapidly and within a week had both the cystostomy tube and Foley catheter removed. He experienced some urinary dribbling but understood that regaining urinary control was a gradual process and was not overly disturbed about it. Mrs. Haynes was pleased that Jerry had come through the surgery so well and would be discharged soon. However, she worried about his sexual potency and thought that he probably did, too.

One morning, almost two weeks after the surgery, Mrs. Haynes was awakened by a telephone call. "Karen, I woke up this morning with an erection," Jerry stated. "I guess everything is going to be all right after all. I'm so relieved!" Karen was also relieved and encouraged by Jerry's good news. For the first time they spoke of the second honeymoon they had been planning before the surgery, and decided to make their cruise reservations for the earliest departure Dr. Raman thought possible.

17 What are the variety of factors that may account for erection in the period after genitourinary surgery?

18 If you were the nurse present during a time when a patient experiences an erection, how do you think you would respond?

25 Identify the physical and psychological elements (both intrapersonal and interpersonal) that would encourage Mr. Haynes's social reintegration and increase his coping abilities in the postoperative period.

PHYSICAL	PSYCHOLOGICAL

26 Health teaching in preparation for discharge is a responsibility of the nurse. What health teaching would you undertake to assist Mr. Haynes in optimal adjustment to home and community?

pecial problem, Family
'0.
'uct survey: urinary
'74 **4**:52-60, Jan.,

man, Donna S.:
of infection,
Fri**1**:2150-2152,

he home,
922-924,

pect

of psychogenic impotence, American Journal of Psychotherapy **27**:421-429, July, 1973.

Hall, Aileen: Nursing care of patient following prostatectomy, Canadian Nurse **64**:35, Dec., 1968.

Jacobson, Linbania: Illness and human sexuality, Nursing Outlook **22**:50-53, Jan., 1974.

Kasselman, Mary Jo: Nursing care of the patient with benign prostatic hypertrophy, American Journal of Nursing **66**:1026-1030, May, 1966.

Morel, Alice: Urethral catheters—an ancient device, RN **35**:40-43, April, 1972.

PART THREE ·
THE PATIENT WITH PSYCHOPHYSIOLOGICAL DYSFUNCTION

THEORETICAL BASE

Nearly 500 years B.C., Socrates returned from military service to report to his Greek countrymen that the Thracian barbarians were, in one respect, in advance of the Greek civilizations, for "they knew that the body could not be cured without the mind." Ignorance of the whole, he believed, accounted for the fact that cures for many diseases were unknown to the physicians of Greece. This idea of a unitary concept, that mind and body are inseparable, infers that each influences the other and that man is an entity and cannot be separated into singularly functioning parts.

The term "psychosomatic" came into common use in the United States about 1935 and was popularly adopted after World War II. It has been widely used and even more widely misinterpreted by those who use it. We have used the term "psychophysiological" interchangeably with "psychosomatic" throughout this section, to imply, in a broad fashion, the simultaneous application of physiological and psychological principles to the study of illness. This approach facilitates the making of definitive diagnoses and the planning and implementation of comprehensive health care. Based on the belief that mind and body are one and that they function as interactive and interdependent organs, psychosomatic medicine aims at discovering the precise nature of the relationship between emotions and bodily function.

Large number of persons seeking health care can benefit from this approach to medical problems. For example, 60% of all patients seen in the office of the family practitioner have accompanying emotional problems. One third of patients with chronic illness fall into this group, and one third of those with acute illness have symptoms that are dependent on emotional factors in part, even though organic findings are present.

105

8 · THE PATIENT WITH PEPTIC ULCER

CLINICAL CASE STUDY

Harriet Bell sat in the x-ray department, waiting. Neither the upper gastro-intestinal series nor the waiting were new to her. In fact, Mrs. Bell was so familiar to everyone in the x-ray department that they all called her by her first name—a familiarity at which she bristled. Not accustomed to being inactive, Mrs. Bell hated to wait for anything. She smiled to herself, wondering why the wait bothered her so much this time. Previously her x-ray studies on an out-patient basis had allowed her to race back to her office immediately. This time she was an inpatient with nothing to race back to, except perhaps a cold, bland breakfast.

Harriet Bell was 38 years old and had a six-year history of recurring duodenal ulcer. Each time her symptoms reappeared, Mrs. Bell was placed on a regimen of rest, diet, and medication. In two to four weeks she felt as good as new and rarely missed a full day at work. This time, however, Dr. Liaros, Mrs. Bell's internist, insisted on hospitalization for supervision of her ulcer regimen and further diagnostic studies. Dr. Liaros knew that Mrs. Bell's life-style was incompatible with the rest and dietary management required for proper healing and prevention of recurring ulcers. Consequently he planned to use this hospitalization to help her understand the complexity of ulcer man-agement and the possible alternatives available to her in maintaining her own health. Dr. Liaros and the health team on the medical unit had instituted teaching conferences for patients with ulcers and planned to include Mrs. Bell in these conferences as soon as the diagnostic work-up was completed.

1 Mrs. Bell disliked the use of her first name by staff members of the x-ray department. Consider the factors that might have influenced her response to such familiarity.

DIAGNOSTIC STUDY	NURSING RESPONSIBILITIES
b. stool for occult blood	
c. gastric analysis (with histamine)	
d. tubeless gastric analysis	
e. gastroscopy	

6 A peptic ulcer occurs because the lining of the stomach or the duodenum has been changed so that it can be eroded. What physiological factors are thought to be responsible for this change?

7 What are the personality correlates and/or emotional predispositions thought to be influencing factors in peptic ulcer formation?

8 Ulcer symptoms vary depending on the location of the ulcer and the individual involved. Which of the following are possible ulcer symptoms?

12 Recent trends in dietary management of ulcer patients lean toward a more liberalized approach. Discuss the advantages of such a regimen.

13 In caring for a patient with an ulcer, the nursing approach is extremely important. Using the chart below, identify the short-term nursing care goals for Mrs. Bell, the rationale for these goals, and appropriate nursing actions.

SHORT-TERM GOALS	RATIONALE	NURSING ACTION

Although hospitalized, Mrs. Bell continued to carry out her job responsibilities. The nursing staff learned that Mrs. Bell owned her own advertising agency and was a highly successful businesswoman. Visitors came and went at all hours of the day and night, and Mrs. Bell's telephone was constantly busy.

Several days after Mrs. Bell's admission, Mrs. Lundine, a patient in the room across the hall, complained to the nursing staff about the noise and activity in and around Mrs. Bell's room, which she compared with the hustle and bustle of an airline terminal. She believed that Mrs. Bell had too many visitors, who stayed too long and were too loud. She found the frequent ringing of the telephone, which disturbed her attempts to rest, annoying and requested that some action be taken.

14 Mrs. Lundine ended her complaint by saying: "It's not fair that some people get away with everything and break the rules all the time. I don't think I can stand the noise any longer. Something needs to be done about her." Which response to Mrs. Lundine is likely to be the most helpful initially?

1. "I can appreciate how troublesome this must be for you. I'll talk it over with the other nurses and see what solutions we can come up with."
2. "We don't expect her to be a patient on this floor much longer. Her doctor will let her go home as soon as her symptoms clear up."
3. "Everyone bends the rules a little bit in one way or another. Your granddaughter comes to visit and she's only 5 years old."

18 Nursing intervention could involve Mrs. Bell in direct or indirect ways. Identify direct and indirect actions that could be taken to facilitate the resolution of this problem.

DIRECT ACTIONS	INDIRECT ACTIONS

19 What are the advantages and disadvantages of involving Mrs. Bell in direct or indirect ways?

ADVANTAGES	DISADVANTAGES
a. direct involvement	
b. indirect involvement	

20 Use the guide below to formulate a verbal approach to Mrs. Bell regarding Mrs. Lundine's complaints.

DYNAMICS	RATIONALE FOR INTERVENTION
VERBAL APPROACH	**POSSIBLE OUTCOMES**

23 Although some staff members viewed Mrs. Bell as uncooperative and aloof, others viewed her as a successful woman to be admired. In terms of each polar position, how would you expect these staff members to respond to Mrs. Bell?

MRS. BELL AS AN UNCOOPERATIVE PERSON	MRS. BELL AS A PERSON TO BE ADMIRED

24 What are your suggestions for how the nursing staff could resolve the problem of their conflicting views of Mrs. Bell?

25 It is believed that persons who have peptic ulcer frequently have unmet dependency needs. How does this fit with the behavior Mrs. Bell has exhibited and the information you have about her?

26 Review the Janis framework of anticipatory fear described on pp. 4 and 5. At which fear level would you place Mrs. Bell?

Why?

27 During the conference with Mr. Bell, he shared with the staff Mrs. Bell's feelings of dehumanization during this hospital experience. What practices, events, or circumstances are dehumanizing to hospitalized patients, and

FEAR-AROUSING STATEMENT	FEAR-REDUCING STATEMENT
a. smoking	a. smoking
b. eating rich foods	b. eating rich foods
c. drinking alcoholic beverages	c. drinking alcoholic beverages
d. business responsibilities	d. business responsibilities
e. business-related entertaining	e. business-related entertaining

30 Incorporating what you have learned in the preceding questions, identify the long-term nursing care goals for Mrs. Bell, the rationale for these goals, and appropriate nursing actions.

on the patient, Nursing Clinics of North America **5:**715-724, Dec., 1970.

Hays, Dorothea R.: Waiting: a concept in nursing. In Burd, Shirley F., and Marshall, Margaret A., editors: Some clinical approaches to psychiatric nursing, New York, 1963, The Macmillan Co., pp. 67-72.

Levine, Myra E.: The intransigent patient, American Journal of nursing **70:**2106-2111, Oct., 1970.

Purintun, Lynn R., and Nelson, Louella, I.: Ulcer patient: emotional emergency, American Journal of Nursing **68:**1930-1933, Sept., 1968.

Spitzer, Stephen P., and Volk, Barbara A.: Altercasting the difficult patient, American Journal of Nursing **71:**732-735, April, 1971.

roommate urged her to seek medical attention. At that point Evelyn was not only too weak to argue but willing to go to the student health service on campus.

Evelyn was favorably impressed by the student health workers. A student nurse elicited a complete history from her before she was examined by a medical student/nursing student team under the guidance of an attending physician. A medical technology student performed a venipuncture and drew 10 ml. of blood, after which an intravenous infusion was begun. Evelyn was assigned a private room in the infirmary and given sedation intramuscularly. She drifted off to sleep while worrying if she'd be well enough to get home for part of the week-end.

Evelyn's symptoms subsided rapidly, and in two days she was discharged from the infirmary. She was given an appointment for diagnostic studies on an outpatient basis at University Hospital and instructed to get plenty of rest and continue on a low-residue diet. The team in the student health service scheduled a follow-up visit in two weeks, after the results of Evelyn's diagnostic studies would be available.

1 The diagnostic studies ordered for Evelyn were proctoscopy and barium enema. Discuss the nature of each test and the nursing responsibilities involved in preparing patients for such tests.

DIAGNOSTIC STUDY	NURSING RESPONSIBILITIES
a. proctoscopy	
b. barium enema	

2 Evelyn was diagnosed as having ulcerative colitis. As a member of the team in the student health service responsible for developing a teaching plan for Evelyn, what should you know about ulcerative colitis before you talk with her? Use the format below.
a. etiology

b. incidence

121

OVERALL APPROACH	POSSIBLE OUTCOMES

6 Incorporating what you have learned in the preceding questions, formulate a teaching plan for Evelyn, using the guide below.

HEALTH TEACHING	RATIONALE

7 Nursing intervention could involve Mr. and Mrs. Feldman in direct or indirect ways. Identify direct and indirect actions that could be taken to involve Evelyn's parents in promoting and maintaining Evelyn's health.

DIRECT ACTIONS	INDIRECT ACTIONS

123

sexual views. These exacerbations were effectively controlled with brief periods of confinement in the infirmary, rest, medication, and diet.

Evelyn and Steve planned to marry after graduation from college. Steve was looking into graduate schools in other states, and Evelyn was torn between the excitement of moving away with Steve and leaving her parents. Her parents took the news of her anticipated marriage better than she expected and welcomed Steve cordially each time she brought him home. However, Evelyn could not help but think that their outward acceptance of her future plans was predicated on their fear that Evelyn's colitis symptoms would recur if they responded openly and honestly.

12 In the medical management of ulcerative colitis a variety of medications may be used. What is the purpose of each of the following types of drugs? What are the nursing responsibilities involved?

PURPOSE	NURSING RESPONSIBILITIES
a. antiemetics	
b. sedative-antispasmodics	
c. oral or parenteral minerals	
d. vitamin supplements	
e. steroids	
f. sulfonamides	

NURSING CARE	RATIONALE

17 What circumstances do you believe were influential in the exacerbation of Evelyn's symptoms?

18 It is believed that individuals with ulcerative colitis have similar histories regarding significant losses. What past, present, and anticipated future losses are relevant for Evelyn?

PAST LOSSES	PRESENT LOSSES	ANTICIPATED FUTURE LOSSES

Dr. Nancy Sebastiano, the internist managing Evelyn's care, was extremely concerned that Evelyn's condition deteriorated despite medical treatment. She continued to lose weight and became extremely weak, withdrawn, and apathetic.

Dr. Carlton Lechner, a surgeon, was called in by Dr. Sebastiano to assess Evelyn's problems. After a thorough review of the x-ray and laboratory studies and a complete physical examination, he recommended total colectomy with ileostomy for Evelyn. He suggested efforts to improve Evelyn's overall condition prior to surgery so that operative risk would be reduced to a minimum.

Dr. Sebastiano spoke with Evelyn and her parents about Dr. Lechner's findings. She discussed with them the reasons for performing ileostomy, the advantages of a one-stage procedure, and the expected postoperative course after such surgery. She verbalized the thoughts she believed the Feldmans could not express concerning the sociocultural significance of elimination. Dr. Sebastiano consulted with Evelyn about the preoperative preparation she believed important. In addition to intensive efforts to improve Evelyn's general physical health, Dr. Sebastiano encouraged her to think about working with a mental health counselor. She also mentioned arranging for a visit from a young woman who had previ-

BEFORE SURGERY	AFTER SURGERY

Dr. Lechner came immediately from surgery to tell the Feldmans and Steve that Evelyn had successfully undergone total colectomy and ileostomy. He explained that he had placed a temporary appliance over the ileostomy stoma for collection of ileostomy drainage to prevent excoriation of peristomal skin. "The ileostomy will probably function within 12 to 24 hours and may discharge a large amount of liquid fecal matter. Don't be surprised if this happens," Dr. Lechner stated.

Evelyn didn't remember a great deal about her immediate postoperative period. She did recall the tubes—it seemed as though she had a tube everywhere. The tube in her nose was particularly annoying, and the discomfort in her nose and throat frequently woke her from her dozings. The deep-breathing and coughing exercises were particularly difficult because of the nasogastric tube. Each breath and cough caused the tube to move and increased the irritation in Evelyn's throat.

Evelyn was ambulated on her first postoperative day. Two days later her nasogastric tube and Foley catheter were removed and oral fluids were initiated. She tolerated the institution of oral fluids well, and after laboratory confirmation of her good fluid and electrolyte status, the intravenous fluids were discontinued.

Although some aspects of Evelyn's postoperative recovery were encouraging to the health care team, other aspects were creating difficulties. Evelyn hated the odor from her ileostomy bag and could not bear the sight of her stoma. She covered her eyes each time the bag was changed and the peristomal skin cleansed. She had frequent periods of depression, and the nursing staff often described her as silent and apathetic. Whenever efforts were made to involve Evelyn in the care of her ileostomy, she stated that she was "too weak to learn today."

The Feldmans voluntarily met several times with the mental health counselor to discuss how they could best support Evelyn during this difficult time in her life. They were particularly concerned about Steve's negative reaction to Evelyn's surgery and its effect on their daughter. He refused to talk with the mental health counselor despite encouragement from them. The Feldmans realized the situation was difficult for Steve, too, but were not prepared when he broke his engagement to Evelyn.

23 What nursing measures can you undertake to relieve Evelyn's discomfort from her nasogastric tube? Include rationale.

NURSING MEASURES	RATIONALE

29 As expected with young persons undergoing colectomy, depression is the initial response? Why?

30 What behavior patterns of hospitalized persons would indicate depression?

31 What nursing actions could be helpful to combat depression?

32 What are anatomical and physiological changes resulting from colectomy that may adversely influence sexual performance, and what are the purely psychosocial factors?

ANATOMICAL/PHYSIOLOGICAL CHANGES	PSYCHOSOCIAL FACTORS

33 The value an individual has as an attractive sexual person often lies in the eyes of the partner. Consider how the surgery may have affected Steve's perception of Evelyn's sexual attractiveness.

34 Consider how Steve's response may have affected Evelyn's feelings about her own sexual attractiveness.

NURSING ACTION	RATIONALE

38 Incorporating what you have learned in the preceding questions, identify short-term and long-term nursing care goals for Evelyn, the rationale for these goals, and appropriate nursing actions.

GOALS	RATIONALE	NURSING ACTION
a. short-term		
b. long-term		

Evelyn was measured for a permanent ileostomy appliance ten days after her surgery. She found this new appliance much easier to apply than the bags she had been wearing and began to take interest in self-care. The nursing staff encouraged her in her efforts to become more independent and offered reassurance when difficulties arose. Drs. Lechner and Sebastiano consulted with the health team about discharge planning and referral to a community health agency.

39 Health teaching in preparation for discharge is a responsibility of the nurse. What health teaching would you undertake to assist Evelyn in optimal adjustment to home and community?

10 · THE PATIENT WITH RHEUMATOID ARTHRITIS

CLINICAL CASE STUDY

Leonard Pauley was worried. He took pride in the job he did and wondered how much longer his reputation as one of the fastest and best assembly line workers in the plant would survive. Recently he had noticed tenderness and swelling in the joints of his fingers, wrists, and elbows and woke up in the mornings with generalized muscular aching and fatigue. His work was beginning to show the effects, and the guys were kidding him about "old age creeping up."

Alice, Leonard's wife, was also worried. She feared losing the things for which they had strived so hard and for which she had pushed Leonard all their married years. It had taken them both several years of scrimping and saving to buy the things they now possessed. Their new house was Alice's dream come true, and even though they had lived in it for almost a year, she made sure that it always looked like a model home. It belied the fact that a family with two children and one large dog resided beneath its roof.

Having the full responsibility for the children while Leonard worked two jobs was difficult for her and for the children, who missed a closeness with their father. However, all the hard work and frustration culminated in achieving their present comfortable level of living. Alice couldn't bear the thought that Leonard might be ill and unable to continue working.

Alice and Leonard were both 42 years old. Twenty years of marriage brought with it one son, Lenny, age 18 years, and a daughter, Cynthia, age 15 years. The Pauleys vividly remembered their early years together, which were extremely difficult financially. Now things were looking up. They had a new house and a new car, and were planning to send Lenny to the local community college. Leonard didn't want his son to be a manual laborer as he was and hoped Lenny would be a professional man.

As his symptoms progressed, Leonard decided to seek medical care. He stopped in the health office at work and requested to see the plant physician. During the initial history the industrial nurse noted the enlarged, stiff joints of Leonard's hands. She was not surprised when Dr. Abbassi gave a diagnosis of rheumatoid arthritis. Dr. Abbassi also discussed with Leonard the value of hospitalization for further diagnosis and treatment.

4 Of what value are the sedimentation rate and latex fixation test in patients with rheumatoid arthritis?

5 Mr. Pauley's symptoms worsened, and his fingers, wrists, and elbows became exquisitely tender. He also complained of discomfort in his ankles and feet. What nursing measures can you undertake to relieve Mr. Pauley's discomfort? Include rationale.

NURSING MEASURES	RATIONALE

6 In the medical management of rheumatoid arthritis a variety of medications may be used. What is the purpose of each of the following types of drugs? What are the nursing responsibilities involved?

	PURPOSE	NURSING RESPONSIBILITIES
a. salicylates		
b. anti-inflammatory drugs		
c. steroids		
d. antimalarial compounds		

Continued.

137

to assign someone so incompetent to his care, or he would bring suit against the entire hospital.

In the meantime, Mrs. Pauley began to call Mary Files daily to ask when Leonard could be discharged and return to work. When she visited, she cornered whomever of the nursing staff was available and spoke at great length about the extreme financial difficulty the family would suffer if Leonard couldn't work.

Mary Files realized the situation was entirely out of hand. Her staff disappeared when they saw Mrs. Pauley coming, and Mary herself groaned at each daily phone call. The staff avoided Mr. Pauley at exercise time, thereby simultaneously avoiding his outbursts, accusations of incompetence, and threats to bring suit. Mary called for a nursing team conference to problem-solve and develop a realistic plan of care for Mr. Pauley.

9 It is believed that persons who have rheumatoid arthritis frequently have chronically inhibited rage. How does this fit with the behavior Mr. Pauley has exhibited and the information you have about him?

10 Certain elements are important in evaluating the significance of body image or its alteration. Which of the following are true?
   a. That which is acquired later in life has greater emotional significance than that which occurs earlier in life.
   b. That which occurs abruptly is far more traumatic than that which develops gradually.
   c. That which involves the external genitalia and the reproductive organs is more threatening than that which does not.
   d. That which is internal and cannot be viewed by the patient is more disturbing emotionally than conditions which are evident.
   1. a, b, c   3. a, d
   2. b, c   4. all of the above

11 Mr. Pauley was experiencing a change in the structure of his face and the structure and function of his hand. What do you know about the significance of body image and its alteration, both in general and specifically in Mr. Pauley's case? How can you use this knowledge to plan for Mr. Pauley's care?

KNOWLEDGE BASE	NURSING ACTION

17 On the basis of the rationales you have determined, would you reformulate your initial verbal response? If so, return to question 13 to reassess your answers.

18 Assuming that Mary Files wanted to respond with each of the five following intentions to Mr. Pauley when he told her never again to assign someone so incompetent to his care, or he would sue the entire hospital, write down what she might have said.

a. evaluating _____

_____

_____

_____

b. interpreting _____

_____

_____

_____

c. probing _____

_____

_____

_____

d. reassuring _____

_____

_____

_____

e. understanding _____

_____

_____

_____

19 Which of the above responses are likely to be the most appropriate to the circumstances?

25 In this instance, it was Mr. Pauley, the patient, who initiated open communication about what he had overheard. However, other patients might respond in different ways. Identify other responses and how they might influence the course of an individual's hospitalization.

POSSIBLE RESPONSE	INFLUENCE ON HOSPITALIZATION

26 Identify the physical and psychological elements that would encourage Mr. Pauley's social reintegration and increase his coping abilities.

PHYSICAL	PSYCHOLOGICAL

27 Mrs. Pauley frequently conveyed her belief to the nursing staff that Leonard seldom expressed interest in and affection for Lenny and Cynthia. The staff noted that neither child visited Mr. Pauley more than once a week and that the visits were very brief. There were no outward displays of affection on any of these occasions. The staff discussed referral of the Pauley family to a family counseling agency. Do you think this would be helpful? If so, why? If not, why not?

28 What actions would be important in assisting Mrs. Pauley and the children with their own personal adjustments? What might be required of them in helping Mr. Pauley? What are the rationales for the actions recommended?

31 Heat treatments are of great value in the care of a patient with rheumatoid arthritis. What can you teach Mr. Pauley about the rationale for use of heat and the ways he can apply heat in his own home or place of work?

RATIONALE	METHODS OF HEAT APPLICATION

32 Health teaching in preparation for discharge is a responsibility of the nurse. What other health teaching would you undertake to assist Mr. Pauley in optimal adjustment to home and community?

Mary Files had talked with Lee Ehrenreich, Leonard's foreman, on the phone several times. During nursing rounds one afternoon she met Mr. Ehrenreich in Leonard's room. "We have transferred Leonard to our plant security department," he stated. "I sure hate to lose Leonard on the assembly line. He's my best worker. However, our nurse and doctor feel it's a good move for Leonard."

"I'm pleased about it," Leonard stated. "Although I, too, hate to leave Lee and the other guys, I'm glad I can still work somewhere. Wait until Alice and the kids hear. I'm going to call and tell them right now!"

REFERENCES

Brower, Phyllis, and Hicks, Dorothy: Maintaining muscle function in patients on bedrest, American Journal of Nursing **72:**1250-1253, July, 1972.

Gould, Robert: Measuring masculinity by the size of a paycheck, Ms. **1:**18-21, June, 1973.

Loxley, Alice K.: The emotional toll of crippling deformity, American Journal of Nursing **72:**1839-1840, Oct., 1972.

Marmor, Leonard, Walike, Barbara C., and Upshaw, Mary Jane: Rheumatoid arthritis: surgical intervention, American Journal of Nursing **67:**1430-1433, July, 1967.

Murray, Ruth L. E.: Body image development in adulthood, Nursing Clinics of North America **7:**617-630, Dec., 1972.

Murray, Ruth L. E.: Principles of nursing intervention for the adult patient with body image changes, Nursing Clinics of North America **7:**697-707, Dec., 1972.

Olson, Edith V.: The hazards of immobility, American Journal of Nursing **67:**779-797, April, 1967.

Thomas, Mary Durand: Anger in nurse-patient interactions, Nursing Clinics of North America **2:**737-745, 1967.

Walike, Barbara C.: Rheumatoid arthritis: personality factors, American Journal of Nursing **67:**1427-1430, July, 1967.

Walike, Barbara C., Marmor, Leonard, and Upshaw, Mary Jane: Rheumatoid arthritis, American Journal of Nursing **67:**1420-1426, July, 1967.

Williams, R. L., and Krasnoff, A. G.: Body image and physiological patterns in patients with peptic ulcer and rheumatoid arthritis, Psychosomatic Medicine **26:**701-709, 1964.

STUDENT AND INSTRUCTOR GUIDE

This student and instructor guide provides specific answers to the multiple-choice questions in the clinical case studies and general responses or suggestions for responses to the other questions.

The guide was designed purposefully as part of the text, rather than as a separate answer book for the instructor alone, because of our conviction that the answers to the questions and the suggestions for responses also belong to the student. It offers an opportunity for instant feedback, an important but frequently violated principle of learning.

The student, by using the reference lists that accompany each clinical case study, can refer to appropriate sources for validation or correction and/or further theoretical information. The opportunity to do so is, we believe, an important element in the process of socialization into a profession that demands adequate decision-making skills. Taking advantage of this opportunity is one of the hallmarks of an inquiring mind.

PART ONE • THE PATIENT EXPERIENCING ANXIETY

1 • Three preoperative patients

1. 3
2. 3
3. 2
4. 4
5. 2
6. 1
7. 1
8. 2
9. 1
10. a. Cleanse the skin.
    b. Remove hair that harbors bacteria.
11. Areas to be prepared will vary according to surgical approach and hospital policy; however, suggestions are:
    a. abdominal surgery
       (1) upper—nipple line to, but not including, pubic area and from bed line to bed line
       (2) lower—below nipple line, to, and including pubic area and from bed line to bed line
    b. chest surgery—chest and back from sternum to spine on affected side, including shoulder and upper arm
    c. perineal surgery—below umbilicus to and including pubic and perineal areas and upper thighs, anterior and posterior
12. To ensure maximum protection from bacterial invasion and to allow for extension of the incision if necessary.
13. Have you considered the effects of anxiety on vital signs, pupil size, skin characteristics, digestion, bowel and bladder elimination, appetite, characteristics of speech, motor activity and patterns of rest, relaxation, and sleep?
14. 1
15. 4
16. 2
17. 2
18. 1

muted light and sound may give rise
to sensory distortion or misperception?

5. Preservation of full range of motion of
each joint; prevention of contractural
deformities of the joints and adaptive
shortening of the muscles; maintenance of muscle tone and improvement in venous and lymphatic flow.

6. Each joint in the body: shoulder,
forearm and elbow, wrist, fingers, hip,
knee, ankle, toes.

7.
6 a.	9 e.	11 h.	3 k.	
5 b.	7 f.	12 i.	2 l.	
10 c.	8 g.	4 j.	1 m.	
10 d.				

8. 4
9. 3
10. Have you considered Mrs. Cameron's
wishes as well as Jon's and Linda's
personal beliefs, coping abilities, and
financial state?
11. Have you considered the pros and
cons of *each* side of the question?
12. 2

13. 4
14. 3
15. 1
16. 3
17. Have you considered aspects of both
the instrumental and expressive roles?
18. Have you considered the desirability
of providing information prior to the
decision-making process and the method and manner in which such information may be given?
19. Have you considered the interactional
aspects of all these factors and the
effects they may have on the partici-
pants?
20. It assists with grief work and movement toward resolution of the mourning process by providing opportunities
to discuss the loss and its significance,
and it sets the stage for movement
from shock and disbelief into developing awareness.
21. Nurses seldom have the opportunity
to attend the wake or the funeral.
Assisting with postmortem care may
serve a similar purpose.

PART TWO • THE PATIENT WITH ALTERATIONS IN BODY IMAGE

4 • The amputee

1. 3
2. 2
3. Have you considered maintenance of
airway, control of hemorrhage, provision of adequate blood volume, assessment of level of consciousness, and
support of homeostatic mechanisms?
4. 4
5. Relevant options are a, b, and c because intermittent claudication usually
occurs after exercise; atrophy, ulceration, and gangrene occur with pro-
longation of arterial impairment.
6. 4
7. Have you considered assessment of
Gary's psychological state, prior surgical experiences, determination of
teaching priorities in terms of prevention of complications, and involvement
of persons Gary would view as supportive?
8. a. Femoral
artery
b. Profunda
artery of
thigh
c. Profunda
artery of
thigh
d. Anterior
tibial
recurrent
artery
e. Anterior
tibial
artery
f. Fibula

g. Tibia
h. Dorsalis
pedis
artery
i. Superior
gluteal
artery
j. Inferior
gluteal
artery
k. Femur
l. Popliteal
artery
m. Anterior
tibial
artery
n. Posterior
tibial
artery
o. Peroneal
artery
p. Posterior
tibial
artery

9. a. Débridement—removal of foreign
bodies, infected and devitalized tissue from a wound.
b. Transection—a cutting completely
through from side to side.
10. Checking of peripheral pulses and of
color and temperature of extremity;
assessment of blood return after compression of nail bed; measures to prevent decreased circulation to the part,
such as elimination of tight dressings
and bedclothes.
11. 3
12. Have you correctly interpreted the
significance of Gary's comments in

149

support of circulation, prevention of swelling, molding of muscles for prosthetic application, and health teaching activities? Have you also noted the differences in anchoring the bandage, contracture problems, etc., with mid-thigh and mid-calf bandaging?

37. Does your answer include position of wheelchair and bed, locking of wheels of wheelchair and bed, body mechanics of patient and nurse, safety factors, and possible collaboration with the physical therapist?

38. Does your answer include exercises in preparation for crutch walking, selection of proper crutches, proper stance, proper gait, safety factors, and collaboration with the physical therapist?

39. Is the extent of the information you offered such that Gary can both understand and implement it? Have you considered what you already know about Gary and what else you need to know in order to be able to help him deal with it?

40. Have you considered the wide range of responses likely?

41. Does your answer take into consideration safety factors at home, rest, exercise, observations to be made and symptoms to be reported, proper care of the stump and prosthesis, information on rental of equipment if needed, necessity for follow-up medical care, and sources of help for possible future problems regarding the masculine role and societal expectations?

5 • The patient undergoing mastectomy

1. Have you considered the value of privacy and communication techniques that encourage verbalization?

2. 2

3. Have you correctly interpreted the significance of Beth's comments in selecting the appropriate response and formulating rationale?

4. Have you considered the communication-inhibiting elements of the remaining responses?

5. 1

6. Have you correctly interpreted the significance of Beth's comments in selecting the appropriate response and formulating rationale?

7. Have you considered the judgmental as well as the communication-inhibiting elements of the remaining responses?

8. Do your answers include sufficient information for use in helping patients understand the differences between each surgical procedure?

9. Have you considered the life-and-death risks involved, as well as the influences of self-concept and body image?

10. 1

11. Deep-breathing and coughing exercises because pressure dressings that tightly encircle the chest make it difficult to breathe deeply and fully expand the lungs.

12. From the background of information you have concerning skin preparation, have you selected the reasons that would impart information without producing a high level of anxiety?

13. For example, a statement of observation that Beth seems close to tears could be made.

14. For example, an open-ended statement of observation encourages verbalization.

15. Have you considered the individuality of each member of this family in terms of psychological orientation, age, sex, and role assumptions? Have you also considered the influences of the family as a system?

16. In addition to the above, have you considered the fact that Beth is involved in both dyadic and group relationships and that the nature and quality of these relationships differ?

17. 2

18. 1

19. Fluids run downhill, and evidence of external bleeding may be found beneath the area of surgery rather than on the dressing itself.

20. A large area of tissue is removed, and many blood vessels and lymph ducts are disrupted.

21. Have you considered muscle tension and venous and lymph drainage?

22. 2

23. 4

24. Have you considered body mechanics, necessary supplies, physiological changes, the need for assistance, and how Beth and Jim can be involved?

25. Have you considered the effects of early ambulation and anatomical and physiological factors in formulating your rationale?

26. 4

27. 4

28. Brushing and combing hair, brushing

lated to Sally's position on CircOlectric bed; perineal hygiene; catheter irrigation; explanation to the patient; and considerations of modesty and privacy?

13. a. First-degree burns involve only the superficial layers of the epidermis; they are characterized by erythema, slight localized edema, muscular discomfort, and tenderness.

b. Second-degree burns vary in depth but are classified as second degree as long as any epithelial elements remain; they are characterized by bright pink, mottled red, or blanched appearance; usually blisters are present and the wound is moist, edematous, and very sensitive.

c. Third-degree burns involve the full thickness of the skin and may involve underlying tissues such as muscle and bone; the burn may appear charred, blanched, or semitranslucent.

14. 1

15. 4

16. Have you considered use of sterile bed linen; reverse isolation; masks, gowns, and gloves; environment of patient unit vs. treatment room or operating room; understanding of surgical aseptic technique; and personnel health?

17. Have you considered administration of pain medication prior to the dressing change, comfortable positioning for both patient and nurse, preplanning and organization, privacy, clear and adequate explanation to the patient, involvement of the patient during the procedure, and the need for emotional support and understanding?

18. Is your answer an open and self-disclosing one, or have you distanced your involvement by answering in a way that you believe is expected of you and that prevents you from acknowledging the reality of a response which may need alteration? If you have not been open, change your answer in this question and in question 19 to reflect your likely response.

19. Have you considered past influences as well as present ones?

20. Statements of observation about what Sally will see as well as other steps to provide anticipatory guidance could be made.

21. Have you considered active and passive, as well as verbal and nonverbal, activities?

22. Anger, depression, anxiety, and repulsion are some examples.

23. Effective nursing care, although patient-centered, should be nurse-controlled so that therapeutic goals can be planned and implemented.

24. 4

25-29. Is your initial verbal response based on an assessment that includes recognition of the nutritional problems common to burn patients, the realistic as well as the feared body image changes that may be anticipated, and their emotional concomitants?

30. Have you considered planning your care around meals; measures to reduce pain, odors, and other deterrents to appetite; determining Sally's food preferences and previous dietary habits; nonhurried atmosphere when feeding; serving hot foods hot and cold foods cold; encouraging Sally to do as much as possible—e.g., cupping her bandaged hands around the glass; self-help eating devices; and distractions such as TV or radio?

31. Your answer should serve as a guide in assessing common positioning needs. Modifications should be made in relation to the individual patient and her particular positioning needs and problems. Remember: no position maintained without change is therapeutic.

32. Knowledge of prefixes and suffixes will aid you in understanding the meaning of many of the terms listed. Most of the definitions are easily available in medical dictionaries or medical-surgical texts. The others are defined for you as follows:

d. Homograft, also called allograft—human skin with a different genotype from the recipient's; usually obtained from cadavers, fresh amputation specimens, and tissue banks.

e. Heterograft, also called xenograft—nonhuman skin, such as porcine skin, used as a substitute for homografts because of greater availability.

f. Isograft—skin taken from one identical twin and given to the other.

g. Autograft—skin taken from, and used on, the patient.

33. Have you considered the interactional effects of the physical and psychological elements you identified? For example, Sally's transfer to the rehabilitation unit exposes her to the

example, urinary dribbling might inhibit or limit social reintegration.

26. Does your answer include importance of fluid intake, continuation of exercises, signs and symptoms to be reported to physician, measures to prevent straining at stool, and limitations on exercise? Have you considered involving Karen in your health teaching activities?

PART THREE • THE PATIENT WITH PSYCHOPHYSIOLOGICAL DYSFUNCTION

8 • The patient with peptic ulcer

1. Have you considered the psychosocial significance of one's name to the individual, as well as its function in terms of privacy and/or interpersonal closeness or distance?
2. Have you considered other responses, such as anger, liking or affection, and increased distance?
3. Have you considered the wide variety of negative meanings that waiting might have for individuals, as well as the less frequent positive meanings? Have you also considered that making someone wait is a means of control?
4. Do your definitions consider the location, age of onset, frequency, socioeconomic level, and predisposing factors in differentiating between each type?
5. Does your answer include sufficient information to adequately prepare a patient for such tests? Do your nursng responsibilities include the actual physical preparation of patients as well as postdiagnostic study observations to be made? Also note the embarrassing aspects of such studies and the need for psychological support.
6. Imbalance between protective and corrosive forces caused by increased tension, irregular dietary habits, inadequate relaxation, and gastrointestinal irritants such as alcohol, coffee, and tobacco.
7. Stress, unmet dependency strivings, and aggression are examples.
8. 4
9. a. Milk neutralizes gastric secretions and delays gastric emptying.
   b. Antacids absorb and neutralize hydrochloric acid; they also coat the stomach. Do your nursing responsibilities include adequate explanation to the patient; diluting or following antacid with water to prevent coating of the esophagus only; and observation for side effects?
10. Anticholinergic drugs block acetylcholine, inhibit gastric secretion of acid and pepsin, block vagal stimulation of smooth muscle, reduce stomach tone and motility, and allow food and antacids time to neutralize gastric acid. Do your nursing responsibilities include adequate explanation to the patient of the purpose of these drugs and observation for side effects?
11. Advantages—have you considered the value to the patient of participation in her own care?
    Disadvantages—have you considered that the patient may view this as rejection?
12. Does your answer consider that a more liberalized approach is less fattening, may decrease the ingestion of large amounts of cholesterol, and is more palatable and, in general, more realistic?
13. Have you considered the importance of information gathering; measures to promote rest and reduce stressful environmental stimuli; efforts to establish a therapeutic relationship; and value of health teaching regarding diet, drugs, and rest?
14. 1
15. It indicates understanding and acceptance and that the situation can be improved.
16. Have you considered the communication-inhibiting elements?
17. In formulating your responses, have you reviewed the types of responses and their definitions on pp. 58 and 59?
18. An example of a direct action would be discussing the situation with Mrs. Bell. An example of an indirect action would be restructuring the environment by relocating Mrs. Bell.
19. In reviewing your answer, would you conclude that it is more appropriate to deal directly with Mrs. Bell rather than around her? However, can indirect involvment be used to complement your direct approach?
20. Have you considered your responses to questions 1, 2, 3, 7, 13, 18, and

155

volved. Information about these classes of drugs is readily available in pharmacological or medical-surgical texts.

13. Does your answer consider the therapeutic goals of such a dietary regimen as well as the need for imagination and ingenuity in motivating Evelyn to eat?

14. Nonvalidated beliefs are a dangerous base for action because it is not known whether the beliefs are founded on fact or not. By not being self-disclosing, Evelyn prevents feedback from her parents that could correct her possible misperception of their feelings.

15. Does your answer consider the individuals and their various interrelationships as well as immediate and long-range actions?

16. In developing your plan of care, have you considered the probable physical problems Evelyn will have, such as frequent stools, dehydration, fever, stomatitis, tenesmus, malaise, weight loss, and pressure areas, as well as the concomitant psychological responses?

17. Have you considered the problems of increased tension, decreased rest, more pressure to succeed, and more potential losses?

18. Have you considered all losses of persons, parts, structures, or functions of the body, as well as psychological status?

19. Have you considered the psychosocial factors?

20. a. Have you considered drug therapy such as steroids and intramuscular iron; improvement of fluid and electrolyte status; dietary management; blood transfusions; comfort measures; and prevention of other problems such as complications of immobility?

  b. Have you considered teaching for prevention of postoperative complications; use of sulfonamides, enemas, and a retention catheter; nasogastric intubation; skin preparation; and thorough explanation for each?

21. By helping her to recognize, anticipate, and prepare for the loss, as well as to cope with it afterward.

22. They can serve supportive and reassuring functions, offer practical everyday advice, and aid in social reintegration.

23. Does your answer consider the possible problems of intubation, such as loss of fluid and electrolytes; irritation, ulceration, and necrosis of the nares; interference with ventilation; and inflammation of the pharynx, larynx, and esophagus? Have you considered oral and nasal hygiene, proper taping of the tube to the face, changes of position, and thorough explanations about the tube and its purposes in your nursing measures?

24. Does your answer include measures designed to support respiration, circulation, and electrolyte balance and to prevent complications? Have you considered management of postoperative pain? Implicit in your answers should be consideration for the approach used by health team members when caring for Evelyn.

25. Have you considered prevention of infection in the incisional area, protection of the peristomal skin, relationship of the healing process to fluid and electrolyte status, reduction of odors, and consistency of nursing approach, to name a few?

26. The stoma is irrefutable evidence of alteration in body image and body function generally viewed as socially unacceptable.

27. Does your answer include statements of observation about what Evelyn will see as well as other steps to provide anticipatory guidance?

28. Have you considered active and passive, as well as verbal and nonverbal, activities?

29. The patient is bereaved and is mourning the loss of a body part, in terms of both function and structure, and possibly status losses as well.

30. Does your answer include behavior patterns that are physiological (e.g., loss of appetite and decreased gastrointestinal motility) as well as psychological (e.g., crying and saddened affect) in nature?

31. Does your answer include measures to combat the physiological as well as the psychological effects of depression?

32. There are relatively few anatomical and physiological changes resulting from colectomy that may adversely influence sexual performance, except in the case of older males who have had abdominal-perineal resection. In these instances some inability to maintain erection has been reported. Prob-

dysfunction on pp. 105 and 106?
Have you abstracted the principles
and applied them specifically in **Mr.**
Pauley's case, based on what you know
about him up to this point?

12. Briefly, the significant persons in **Mr.**
Pauley's life who are likely to have
the potential for influencing his self-
view in either positive or negative di-
rections are: wife, children, parents,
other relatives, friends, co-workers,
and health care personnel in both
work and hospital settings.

13. In formulating your initial verbal response, have you correctly and appropriately assessed the situation by
considering the many elements in, and
components of, Mr. Pauley's response?

14. Is your answer based on a review of
the definitions of intents given on pp.
58 and 59?

15. Is your rationale based on a com-
munication-facilitating element inherent in the intent?

16. Is your rationale based on a communication-inhibiting element inherent in the other intents?

17. Consider your answers in questions
13 to 16 in formulating your response.

18. In formulating your responses have
you reviewed the definitions of intents
given on pp. 58 and 59?

19. Is your answer based on the application of facilitative communication
principles to Mr. Pauley's specific situation?

20. Discord in the marital and family relationship, which is likely to place additional pressure on Mr. Pauley rather
than reduce the strain he is experiencing. It implies that the dynamic
of anger is operant in this relationship.

21. Incorporate the understanding in a
total plan of care and identify the
specific needs and appropriate nursing
actions reflected by the situation.

22. Is your answer an open and self-disclosing one, or have you distanced
your involvement by answering in a
way that you believe is expected of
you but that prevents you from acknowledging the reality of a response
which may need alteration? If you
haven't been open, change your answer in this question and in question
23 to reflect your likely response.

23. Have you considered past influences
as well as present ones?

24. It may influence the course of hospitalization negatively if patients and
nurses respond with mutual withdrawal
or anger and increase their interpersonal distance. It may influence the
course of hospitalization positively if
it encourages future communication
among patients and nurses and de-
creases their interpersonal distance.

25. Does your answer build on your response to question 24?

26. Have you considered the interactional
effects of the physical and psychological elements you identified? For example, should Mr. Pauley develop a
contracture that limits his mobility
even more, his coping ability could
be adversely affected.

27. Counseling is helpful when the par-
ticipants are motivated to engage in
it and to alter their behavior. It
would be helpful for this family to
learn to communicate together and to
move toward a resolution of their difficulties.

28. Does your answer consider the need
for assessment of the quality of adjustment of Mrs. Pauley, Lenny, and
Cynthia, their level of growth and development, and their openness to
health teaching and readiness for nursing intervention?

29. Have you considered the physical
therapist, the plant physician, the industrial nurse, Mr. Pauley's foreman,
the family doctor, and the social
worker, to name a few?

30. Do your short-term goals include developing open communication with
Mr. Pauley, the need for health teaching, maintenance of joint mobility
and muscle tone, promotion of comfort, and efforts toward functional in-
dependence? Do your long-term goals
include both physical and psychological aspects of assisting Mr. Pauley
and his family in their adjustment to
a chronic systemic disease for which
there is no known cure?

31. Heat provides temporary relief of
pain, decrease in joint stiffness and
swelling, and muscle relaxation. Have
you considered tub baths and showers,
hot moist compresses, electric blanket,
and home use of paraffin dips in your
answer?

32. Does your answer include importance
of rest, proper diet for avoidance of
weight gain, good posture, adequate
understanding of management of affected joints, special equipment, and
measures to preserve joint function
and prevent deformities? Do your
health teaching activities include Mrs.
Pauley?